ENDING DISCF
PEOPLE W
SUBSTANCE ⏤⏤ DISORDERS

The Evidence for Stigma Change

Committee on the Science of Changing Behavioral Health Social Norms

Board on Behavioral, Cognitive, and Sensory Sciences

Division of Behavioral and Social Sciences and Education

The National Academies of
SCIENCES · ENGINEERING · MEDICINE

THE NATIONAL ACADEMIES PRESS
Washington, DC
www.nap.edu

THE NATIONAL ACADEMIES PRESS   500 Fifth Street, NW   Washington, DC 20001

This activity was supported by Contract No. HHSP233201400020B between the National Academy of Sciences and the U.S. Department of Health and Human Services/Assistant Secretary for Planning and Evaluation. Any opinions, findings, conclusions, or recommendations expressed in this publication do not necessarily reflect the views of the organization or agency that provided support for the project.

International Standard Book Number-13:   978-0-309-43912-1
International Standard Book Number-10:   0-309-43912-4
Digital Object Identifier: 10.17226/23442

Additional copies of this report are available for sale from the National Academies Press, 500 Fifth Street, NW, Keck 360, Washington, DC 20001; (800) 624-6242 or (202) 334-3313; http://www.nap.edu.

Cover credits: Quantum Field, acrylic on 96" × 96" canvas, courtesy of Michael Halliday ©2011. Photograph provided (high resolution 300 dpi), courtesy of Richard Willes ©2016.

Suggested citation: National Academies of Sciences, Engineering, and Medicine. (2016). *Ending Discrimination Against People with Mental and Substance Use Disorders: The Evidence for Stigma Change.* Washington, DC: The National Academies Press. doi: 10.17226/23442.

The National Academies of
SCIENCES · ENGINEERING · MEDICINE

The **National Academy of Sciences** was established in 1863 by an Act of Congress, signed by President Lincoln, as a private, nongovernmental institution to advise the nation on issues related to science and technology. Members are elected by their peers for outstanding contributions to research. Dr. Ralph J. Cicerone is president.

The **National Academy of Engineering** was established in 1964 under the charter of the National Academy of Sciences to bring the practices of engineering to advising the nation. Members are elected by their peers for extraordinary contributions to engineering. Dr. C. D. Mote, Jr., is president.

The **National Academy of Medicine** (formerly the Institute of Medicine) was established in 1970 under the charter of the National Academy of Sciences to advise the nation on medical and health issues. Members are elected by their peers for distinguished contributions to medicine and health. Dr. Victor J. Dzau is president.

The three Academies work together as the **National Academies of Sciences, Engineering, and Medicine** to provide independent, objective analysis and advice to the nation and conduct other activities to solve complex problems and inform public policy decisions. The Academies also encourage education and research, recognize outstanding contributions to knowledge, and increase public understanding in matters of science, engineering, and medicine.

Learn more about the **National Academies of Sciences, Engineering, and Medicine** at www.national-academies.org.

v

Acknowledgments

This report has been reviewed in draft form by individuals chosen for their experience and expertise in accordance with procedures approved by the Report Review Committee of the National Academies of Sciences, Engineering, and Medicine. The purpose of this independent review is to provide candid and critical comments that will assist the institution in making its published report as sound as possible and to ensure that the report meets institutional standards for objectivity, evidence, and responsiveness to the study charge. The review comments and draft manuscript remain confidential to protect the integrity of the deliberative process.

We thank the following individuals for their review of this report: Mary E. Evans, College of Behavioral and Community Sciences, University of South Florida (emeritus); Jeffrey L. Geller, University of Massachusetts Medical School; Gary L. Kreps, Department of Communication, Center for Health and Risk Communication, George Mason University; Matthew W. Kreuter, Public Health and Health Communication Research Laboratory, The Brown School, Washington University in St. Louis; Bruce G. Link, Department of Sociology, University of California, Riverside; Bernadette Mazurek Melnyk, College of Nursing and College of Medicine, Ohio State University; Richard E. Nisbett, Department of Psychology, University of Michigan; Brian Primack, School of Health Sciences, University of Pittsburgh Medical Center; Jacqueline Tulsky, School of Medicine, University of California, San Francisco (emeritus); and Eduardo Vega, Mental Health Association of San Francisco.

Although the reviewers listed above have provided many constructive comments and suggestions, they were not asked to endorse the conclusions or recommendations, nor did they see the final draft of the report before its release. The review of this report was overseen by John Monahan, University of Virginia School of Law, and Floyd E. Bloom, Molecular and Integrative Neuroscience Department, Scripps Research Institute. Appointed by the Academies, they were responsible for making certain that an independent examination of this report was carried out in accordance with institutional procedures and that all review comments were carefully considered. Responsibility for the final content of this report rests entirely with the authoring committee and the institution.

The committee also thanks a number of individuals who presented important content and contextual information for our consideration as speakers in the phase one workshops: Joan Austin, Indiana University; Kay Cofrancesco, Lung Cancer Alliance; Robert Edwards Whitley, McGill University; Sara Evans-Lacko, King's College, London; Tony Foleno, Ad Council; Helena Hansen, New York University; Mark Hatzenbuehler, Columbia University; Anthony Jorm, University of Melbourne; Nathaniel Kendall-Taylor, The Frameworks Institute; Robin Koval, American Legacy Foundation; Alan I. Leshner, American Association for the Advancement of Science (emeritus); Bruce Link, Columbia University; Joe Powell, Association of Persons Affected by Addiction; Susan Rogers, National Mental Health Consumers' Self-Help Clearinghouse; Joanne Silberner, University of Washington; Peggy Swarbrick, Rutgers University; Janet Turan, University of Alabama, Birmingham; Donna Vallone, American Legacy Foundation; Judith Warner, Center for American Progress; Phill Wilson, Black AIDS Institute; Jay A. Winsten, Harvard University; and Lawrence H. Yang, Columbia University.

The committee extends its appreciation to the following experts in sociology, psychology, public health, and nursing for providing papers that synthesized the evidence base on social norms, beliefs, attitudes, and behaviors related to mental illness and substance use disorders: Andrea Bink, Illinois Institute of Technology; Mark Hatzenbuehler, Columbia University; Bruce Link, Columbia University; Bianca Manago, Indiana University; Jennifer Merrill, Brown University; Peter Monti, Brown University; Matthew Pearson, University of New Mexico; Tracy Pugh, Columbia University; Lindsay Sheehan, Illinois Institute of Technology; Allison Webel, Case Western University; and Larry Yang, Columbia University.

Appreciation is also extended to Barbara Wanchisen, director of the Board on Behavioral, Cognitive, and Sensory Sciences, and Robert M. Hauser, executive director of the Division of Behavioral and Social Sciences and Education, for their leadership, guidance, and oversight of and support for the study; and the project team, Jeanne Rivard, Vanessa Lazar, and Renée L. Wilson Gaines. Finally, we thank the executive office reports staff of the Division of Behavioral and Social Sciences and Education, especially Yvonne Wise and Eugenia Grohman, who provided valuable help with the editing and production of the report, and Kirsten Sampson Snyder, who managed the report review process.

David H. Wegman, *Chair*
Lisa M. Vandemark, *Study Director*
Committee on the Science of
Changing Behavioral Health Social Norms

Contents

Summary

Improving the lives of people with mental and substance use disorders has been a priority in the United States for more than 50 years. The Community Mental Health Act of 1963 is considered a major turning point in U.S. efforts to improve behavioral health care. It ushered in an era of optimism and hope and laid the groundwork for the consumer movement and new models of recovery. The consumer movement gave voice to people with mental and substance use disorders and brought their perspectives and experience into national discussions about mental health. The first-hand experiences they shared were often narratives of recovery and social reintegration.

As mental health treatment began to shift from the hospital to the community, recovery became a goal or desired outcome of treatment. Recovery, in this context, is not synonymous with a cure; it is a personal process of movement toward a meaningful, purposeful, and satisfying life. The consumer movement stressed self-empowerment and provision of recovery-oriented support programs run by people with mental and substance use disorders (peer programs). Today, trained peer specialist service programs are integrated into community mental health services, and helping others is a recognized component of recovery. Within the stakeholder community, there are differences of opinion about the risks and benefits of professionalizing this grassroots component of behavioral health care through certification or other standardized processes of education and testing.

Consumer perspectives and the concept of recovery challenged some of the traditional values of the U.S. mental health system, and differences of opinion continue to divide the community of mental health stakeholders across several domains, including diagnosis, treatment, and rights and services, notably as these relate to the needs of people with serious mental illness.[1]

More recent national efforts to improve the lives and safeguard the rights of people with mental and substance use disorders include the 1990 Americans with Disabilities Act (ADA), the 1999 Surgeon General's Report on Mental Health, the ADA Amendments Act of 2008 that expanded protections under the ADA, the Mental Health Parity and Addiction Equity Act of 2008, and protections included in the Affordable Care Act of 2010, as well as other federal-level disability nondiscrimination laws.

Over the same 50-year period, positive change in American public attitudes and beliefs about mental and substance use disorders has lagged behind these advances. "Stigma" is used in the peer-reviewed literature and by the general public to refer to a range of negative attitudes, beliefs, and behaviors. The term stigma itself has been targeted for change by some stakeholder groups, and the Substance Abuse and Mental Health Services Administration (SAMHSA) is moving away from use of this term. In this report, the word stigma and its variants are used, except where the report discusses a more specific dimension of stigma such as prejudicial beliefs or discriminatory practices.

There are considerable gaps in the evidence base on the relationships among behavioral disorders, violence, suicide, and guns, as well as gaps in knowledge about effective policies to reduce gun violence and suicide. Studies have shown that there is a greater relative risk of violence in people with mental illness than in those without mental illness, but the risk is actually very small. Moreover, people with mental illness are more likely to be victims than perpetrators of crime. The risk of violence is greater for people with schizophrenia, bipolar disorder, co-occurring substance use disorder, and those exposed to certain socioeconomic factors, such as poverty, crime victimization, early life trauma, and living in a neighborhood with a high crime rate. Higher incidences of violence are observed in people with substance use disorders and antisocial personality disorders than in people with other psychiatric disorders. The risk of suicide as another form of violence is increased by concurrent substance use; symptoms such as hopelessness and depression; psychotic disorders; bipolar disorder; and environmental factors, such as access to guns and media reports of suicide.

Stigma is not a problem that affects only a few. Most estimates agree

---

[1]Serious mental illness is defined as mental illness resulting in serious functional impairment that substantially interferes with or limits one or more major life activities.

that roughly 1 in 4 or 1 in 5 Americans will experience a mental health problem or will misuse alcohol or drugs during their lifetime. In 2014, nearly 44 million Americans aged 12 and older experienced a mental health problem, and for almost 10 million adults, this was a serious mental illness that met standard diagnostic criteria. In 2013, 17 million adults said that they were misusing or dependent on alcohol, and 24 million people over the age of 12 said that they had used illicit drugs during the prior month. Furthermore, many people are not getting the treatment they may need. Of the 28 million Americans in 2013 who needed treatment for a problem related to alcohol and drugs (that is, met diagnostic criteria), fewer than 1 in 10 received any treatment.

As part of national efforts to understand and change attitudes, beliefs, and behaviors that can lead to stigma and discrimination, the Office of the Assistant Secretary for Planning and Evaluation and SAMHSA of the U.S. Department of Health and Human Services asked the National Research Council and Institute of Medicine to undertake a study of the science of stigma change. In response to that request, the Committee on the Science of Changing Behavioral Health Social Norms was set up under the Board on Behavioral, Cognitive, and Sensory Sciences. The committee was asked to review and discuss evidence on (1) the change in behavioral health norms needed to support individuals with mental and substance use disorders to seek treatment and other supportive services; (2) discrimination, negative attitudes, and stereotyping faced by individuals with mental or substance use disorders; and (3) public knowledge about behavioral health, including how to seek help for people with such disorders.

After reviewing a broad range of available evidence about what works to decrease stigma and to promote affirming attitudes and behaviors, the committee developed recommendations for SAMHSA's Office of Communications and Center for Behavioral Health Statistics and Quality in the areas of communications science and stigma research. The committee also offers a set of conclusions and recommendations about successful stigma change campaigns, how best to encourage people to seek treatment and supportive services for themselves or others, and the research needed to inform and evaluate these efforts in the United States.

PUBLIC KNOWLEDGE AND NORMS

In 1950, the first major national study of public stigma was launched followed by three congressionally mandated studies in 1955, 1956, and 1976 that documented an extreme lack of public knowledge about the nature and causes of mental illness and a deep unwillingness to discuss mental illness. More current public attitudes have been captured through recent population-based surveys, including data from five modules in the General Social Survey fielded between 1996 and 2006 that focused on stigma of mental illness as it is reflected in stereotypes, help- or treatment-seeking, and behavioral dispositions toward people with mental and substance use disorders (how people thought they would behave).

From 1996 to 2006, the stigma associated with mental health treatment decreased, and support for treatment-seeking increased among the general public. More than 80 percent of adults agreed that treatment is effective, and those living in states with higher per capita expenditures on mental health services were more likely to agree that treatment is effective and more likely to report that they had received mental health treatment. By 1996, public knowledge had increased such that respondents differentiated between "problems of daily living" and standard psychiatric disorders. Stigma levels for the former decreased between 1996 and 2006 but stigma related to psychiatric disorders remained high. In 2006, stigma against children and adolescents was lower than that for adults, but nearly one-third of respondents said they would not want their child to befriend a child with depression. One-half of all adult respondents said that treatment would result in discrimination and long-term negative effects on a child's future. Also of importance, despite this large body of evidence on public attitudes, little is known about the relationship between attitudes and actual behaviors toward people with mental and substance use disorders.

In comparing these results to the earlier surveys from the 1950s, researchers found that public knowledge about mental and substance use disorders has increased, specifically concerning the neurobiological underpinnings of mental illness. At the same time, however, beliefs about the underlying causes of substance use disorders have shifted away from the idea of illness in the direction of blame. There is greater public awareness of the stigma associated with both mental and substance use disorders yet public stigma persists at a high level. Data show marked differences across behavioral health conditions: schizophrenia and substance use disorders are more highly stigmatized than other mental disorders; few stigma studies focus specifically on substance use disorders. Perceptions about the dangerousness and unpredictability of people with mental and substance use disorders have increased over time.

CONSEQUENCES OF STIGMA

Stigma is a dynamic multidimensional, multilevel phenomenon that occurs at three levels of society—structural (laws, regulations, policies), public (attitudes, beliefs, and behaviors of individuals and groups), and self-stigma (internalized negative stereotypes). A hallmark of stigma, like stereotyping, is that it overgeneralizes. People who have mental or substance use disorders do not form a discrete, static, or homogeneous group. These disorders can vary among individuals and across a person's lifespan by factors including symptom type and severity. For example, a substance use disorder may be characterized by misuse or chemical dependency, and mental illness may be experienced by an individual as an acute, intermittent, or chronic illness.

Structural stigma exists in public and private institutions, including businesses, the courts, government at all levels, professional groups, school systems, social service agencies, and universities. Stigma at the structural level can appear to endorse discrimination, which contributes to public and self-stigma. Examples include limits on exercising one's civil rights, such as serving on a jury or holding a political office, and discriminatory hiring or admissions policies based on stereotypes. People with mental and substance use disorders are overrepresented in the criminal justice system, which is both a consequence and a source of stigma.

Public stigma is operationalized through the behaviors of individuals and groups of all kinds in society. Relevant groups include educators, employers, health care providers, journalists, police, judges, policy makers, and legislators. With their broad reach, the media have a strong influence on stigma at every level. Despite ongoing and successful efforts to educate media professionals about behavioral disorders, stereotypes of violently mentally ill people are perpetuated in media and social media reports of incidents of mass violence and in public discourse about mental illness. Social media can be a source of stigma or a means of promoting affirming and inclusive attitudes.

Self-stigma reduces self-efficacy and can discourage people from disclosing their conditions for fear of being labeled and subjected to discrimination. Label avoidance in turn discourages help- and treatment-seeking on the part of people with mental and substance use disorders and their families. This avoidance creates a barrier to early diagnosis and treatment, adding to the heavy social burden of untreated mental and substance use disorders, including chronic disease; costs related to victimization, crime, and incarceration; lost productivity; and premature death.

EVIDENCE-BASED STRATEGIES TO REDUCE STIGMA

Strategies to address stigma related to mental and substance use disorders include, but are not limited to,

- education, such as mental health literacy campaigns;
- protest and advocacy (e.g., letter writing and Twitter campaigns);
- programs that facilitate social contact between people with and without behavioral disorders (contact-based programs);

- contact-based education programs, which combine contact with educational content designed to raise public awareness of selected issues or increase public knowledge about mental and substance use disorders;
- media campaigns delivered over a range of platforms, including traditional and newer social media; and
- peer programs in which people who have disclosed their conditions offer their experience and expertise to individuals and families, programs that range from informal peer-led programs to peer specialized services in health services systems.

Disclosure of one's experience with mental or substance use disorders, which is central to both contact-based programs and peer programs of all types, has both risks (being labeled, experiencing discrimination) and benefits (increased likelihood of receiving treatment, decreased self-stigma, increased feelings of inclusion). Ideally, it is done selectively in an informed, supported, and planned manner.

Contact-based interventions alone and contact-based educational programs have the strongest evidence base for reducing stigma. Educational programs alone are not effective for adults but are effective in changing younger people's attitudes. Communication campaigns can be effective but tend to fail for two reasons: failure to identify well-defined goals and objectives for the campaign and failure to reach the intended audience or audiences in a sustained or adequately frequent manner. Protest and advocacy strategies serve to expand the stakeholder base, garner support, and provide a forum for consensus. Regardless of the type of intervention, anti-stigma strategies have often resulted in both intended and unintended consequences.

CONCLUSIONS AND RECOMMENDATIONS

A National-Level Approach

CONCLUSION: The experiences of the U.S. campaigns related to HIV/AIDS and of anti-stigma campaigns in Australia, Canada, and England demonstrate the need for a coordinated and sustained effort over two or more decades to reduce the stigma associated with mental and substance use disorders.

Norms and beliefs related to behavioral health, such as the stigma associated with mental and substance use disorders, are created and reinforced at multiple levels, including day-to-day contact with affected individuals, organizational policies and practices, community norms and beliefs, the media, and governmental law and policy. A number of private and public organizations are already engaged in anti-stigma and mental health promotion efforts, but because these efforts are largely uncoordinated and poorly evaluated, they cannot provide an evidence base for future national efforts.

HHS

RECOMMENDATION 1: The U.S. Department of Health and Human Services should take the lead responsibility among federal partners and key stakeholders in the design, implementation, and evaluation of a multipronged, evidence-based national strategy to reduce stigma and to support people with mental and substance use disorders.

Relevant stakeholder groups would include the following:

- consumers in treatment for mental and substance use disorders and consumer organizations;
- families and others whose lives are touched by mental illness or substance use disorders, including suicide-attempt survivors and loss survivors;
- relevant private sector leadership, including major employers;
- relevant foundations and nongovernmental organizations;
- advocates and advocacy groups, including civil rights and disability law experts;
- insurance companies and pharmaceutical manufacturers;
- journalists and others in the news media, including public health media experts;
- health and behavioral health care providers and administrators, including protective services and social services providers;
- health professional education institutions and professional associations;
- academic researchers, including suicide prevention experts and researchers;
- law enforcement officials and first responders; and
- representatives of federal, state, and local governments.

Early tasks would include the following:

- Identify a lead organization to serve as convener of stakeholders.
- Promote coordination and engagement across local, state, federal, and nongovernmental groups, including the U.S. Departments of Defense, Health and Human Services, Justice, and Labor, and

relevant stakeholder groups to pool resources and promote evidence-based approaches.

- Evaluate current laws and regulations related to people with mental and substance use disorders to identify opportunities for changes that will support people on the path to recovery.
- Support the development of a strategic plan for research and dissemination of evidence about effective strategies to change social norms related to mental and substance use disorders (see Recommendation 3).
- With the federal agencies and other partners, develop a process of identifying and engaging grassroots efforts in each state to promote the implementation of evidence-based programs and fidelity monitoring of service delivery.
- With the federal agencies, establish a long-term, national monitoring system for stigma and stigma reduction.

Collaboration and Coordination

In 2013, eight federal agencies were identified as having programs to support individuals with mental and substance use disorders—the U.S. Departments of Defense, Education, Health and Human Services, Housing, Justice, Labor, Veterans Affairs, and the Social Security Administration—although their specific mission goals vary. Ongoing and enhanced efforts to coordinate across agencies and programs will improve the effectiveness and extend the reach of these programs. To improve the effectiveness and extend the reach of the federal agencies' programs, there are some ongoing efforts to coordinate across the agencies and their programs.

To maximize desired outcomes, collaborative efforts should eschew "ownership" of programs and include cobranding and resource sharing. SAMHSA's ongoing engagement with stakeholders can support the search for common ground, mutually articulated goals, and shared agendas.

The committee has identified structural stigma and stereotypes of dangerousness and unpredictability as major sources of public and self-stigma. Given the importance of reducing stigma in these areas, early efforts could focus on development of a communications campaign or to target policy and decision makers to challenge specific laws, policies, and regulations that discriminate against people with mental and substance use disorders. Such a campaign could develop evidence-based public service announcements to hold in readiness for tragic events, such as mass violence, suicide by school and college students, and suicide clusters.

CONCLUSION: Changing stigma in a lasting way will require coordinated efforts, based on the best possible evidence, which are supported at the national level and planned and implemented by a representative coalition of stakeholders. Engaging a wide range of stakeholders would facilitate consensus building and provide the support needed to overcome major obstacles to the implementation of effective anti-stigma programs in the United States. Barriers and challenges include, but are not limited to, conflict among major stakeholder groups regarding best practices and priorities, resource constraints, and the need to target multiple audiences with variable perceptions and priorities, as well as shifting priorities at the national level.

RECOMMENDATION 2: The U.S. Department of Health and Human Services should evaluate its own service programs and collaborate with other stakeholders, particularly the criminal justice system and government and state agencies, for the purpose of identifying and eliminating policies, practices, and procedures that directly or indirectly discriminate against people with mental and substance use disorders.

Strategic Planning for Research

The committee defines strategic planning as the process undertaken by an agency or organization to define its future and to develop a detailed plan to guide its path from the current state to its vision for the future.

CONCLUSION: A planning process usually results in the development of a key document that includes a plan to ensure that communication is maintained across all stakeholders. This element is especially relevant for the Substance Abuse and Mental Health Services Administration given the agency's ongoing engagement with many stakeholders and collaborators. A strategic plan can also serve as the basis of comparison for an ongoing plan for iterative effectiveness monitoring.

RECOMMENDATION 3: The Substance Abuse and Mental Health Services Administration should conduct formative and evaluative research as part of a strategically planned effort to reduce stigma.

SAMHSA's ongoing program of research on social norms and communications practices could coordinate with national efforts to achieve common goals and objectives. SAMHSA's Office of Communication's future activities could also be informed and supported by partners and participating stakeholders.

Because change occurs slowly, outcome evaluations need to be multifaceted and sustained to capture both direct and indirect effects, as well as intended and unintended consequences. An evaluation plan should include and support community-based participatory research that is based on the principle of partnership, in which community partners act as co-learners with academic partners rather than helpers or recipients. This approach involves community stakeholders from the outset to define both the change targets and the intervention strategies, as well as in the conduct of the research itself. To inform a national campaign, more in-depth formative and evaluative research is critically needed in three areas: communication strategies, contact-based programs, and the role of peers.

Communication Strategies

Communication science provides a basis for understanding the effects of message features, contents, and platforms on four outcomes: cognitive (e.g., attention and memory), affective (e.g., liking, empathy, and fear), persuasive (e.g., attitude and behavior change), and behavioral (e.g., intents and actions). These effects are not discrete. They depend on characteristics of the target audience or audiences, the media platform, the message source, and the specific content and production features used in the message. For example, in a campaign to counter the stereotype of dangerousness in the wake of a tragic event, relevant audiences would include the media, school officials and teachers, young people, parents, and clergy. Messages would target specific smaller groups and would be designed and delivered with input and support of engaged stakeholders, for example, in donated airtime or volunteered time of high-profile supporters and speakers.

> **CONCLUSION: Best practices in choosing effective messages first require that a communications campaign develop well-defined goals for each specific group targeted. Effective messages can then be tailored to the specific target audience for the defined goals.**

Because of the complexity of designing communication messages, efforts to implement the committee's recommendation on this topic should be informed by the results of formative and evaluative research. Research is necessary both before message concepts are generated and after message concepts are created for testing in the field. The perspectives of people with lived experience of mental and substance use disorders should inform anti-stigma campaigns at every stage, including design, delivery, and evaluation.

RECOMMENDATION 4: To design stigma-reduction messaging and communication programs, the Substance Abuse and Mental Health Services Administration should investigate and use evidence from formative and evaluative research on effective communication across multiple platforms.

Several general features of effective communication programs have been identified by research and can inform the work in the committee's recommendations to SAMHSA:

- Identify specific target groups and specific goals appropriate to each group (e.g., legislators and policy makers, employers and landlords, educators, health care practitioners, and people with mental and substance use disorders).
- Make strong appeals that are relevant and personally consequential to particular audiences, for example, young people or veterans.
- Understand how a particular audience orients to a message and what kinds of cues and styles hold their attention so that the message is absorbed and remembered.
- Know what matters most to a specific target group.

Contact-Based Programs

Mixed-methods research has led to the identification of key elements of successful contact-based programs. Outcome research on contact demonstrates robust effects in pre-post studies and at follow-up. In adults, the efficacy of contact-based programs is greater than that of education programs alone across a range of specific target audiences, such as health professionals, college students, and police, but evidence shows that one-time contact is not as effective as repeated contact. In contrast, education programs are effective in changing stigmatizing attitudes among adolescents.

CONCLUSION: To expand the reach of contact-based programs, efforts will be needed to develop a nationally representative cohort of individuals who have disclosed information about their experiences of mental or substance use disorders. Involvement of those individuals needs to be preceded by the design of programs to aid personal consideration and action on disclosure decisions and of

peer training programs to help people consider the risks and benefits of disclosure.

RECOMMENDATION 5: To decrease public and self-stigma and promote affirming and inclusive attitudes and behaviors targeted to specific groups, the Substance Abuse and Mental Health Services Administration should work with federal partners to design, evaluate, and disseminate effective, evidence-based, contact-based programming.

The Role of Peers

Peers play an essential role in combating stigma, in part because they model personal recovery. Their role is critical in helping individuals to overcome the debilitating forces of self-stigma. Peer support programs and services include social and emotional support, as well as practical support related to quality-of-life decisions, delivered by people with mental and substance use disorders. Peer support has existed since the 1970s, but in 2001, several states began efforts to certify and train the peer specialist workforce. By 2012, 36 states had established such programs, although there is considerable variation in the certification programs across these states. State programs vary in terms of stage of development and certification requirements, including the content and process of training, examination criteria, and requirements for continuing education and recertification.

Most research on the outcomes of peer services has focused on quality-of-life measures. Few data are available about the costs and benefits of these programs, although the research suggests that people who use peer support services are more likely to use other behavioral health services of all kinds, including professional services and prescription drugs, which may lead to improved outcomes. Although more peers are becoming certified, stakeholders disagree about the risks and benefits of professionalizing the role given grassroots origins of peer support in the consumer movement.

CONCLUSION: In the United States, there is no established and accepted set of national or state competencies or standards for peer specialists, such as those that apply to other health professionals at state levels.

Although stakeholders do not agree on the risks and benefits of certification for peer support providers, it may contribute to the quality and outcomes of peer services and facilitate research on the effectiveness of these services across a range of outcomes. Programs need to be appropriately targeted to the audience or audiences and implemented at the relevant geographic level. Components of this effort would include standardization of preparation for peer service providers and development of practice guidelines for referral to and delivery of peer services across agencies and organizations. SAMHSA has taken steps in this direction with its 2009 *Consumer-Operated Service Evidence-Based Practices Toolkit* (Chapter 4) and continues to have an important role to play in the development and dissemination of these products and programs across the nation. The National Federation of Families for Children's Mental Health offers a national certification for parent support providers that could serve as a model for future efforts to expand the reach of high-quality peer support services.

> **RECOMMENDATION 6: The Substance Abuse and Mental Health Services Administration should work with partners to design, support, and assess the effectiveness of evidence-based peer programs to support people with mental and substance use disorders along the path to recovery and to encourage their participation in treatment.**

Development of a national strategy for eliminating the stigma of mental and substance use disorders is a challenging, long-term goal that will require collaboration across federal agencies, support from governments at all levels, and engagement of a broad range of stakeholders. No single agency can implement an effective national strategy, but SAMHSA brings specific and unique strengths including well-established stakeholder relations, commitment to the recovery model, and a history of promotion and implementation of prevention and early intervention strategies. Early objectives of a national strategy will include consensus building across a range of issues, design of cost-sharing arrangements, development and implementation of a research strategy including a system for monitoring change in public attitudes, and mechanisms for disseminating information to inform future anti-stigma interventions.

1

Introduction

CONTEXT FOR THE STUDY

Across the United States at any given time, there are hundreds if not thousands of projects and programs aimed at reducing negative attitudes, beliefs, and behaviors concerning mental and substance use disorders, yet stigma persists (Pescosolido et al., 2010; Phelan et al., 2000; Schnittker, 2008); and people with these disorders continue to face prejudice and discrimination in many areas of civic life.[1] To inform future anti-stigma efforts in the United States, this report describes the changes needed to improve the lives of people with mental and substance use disorders and reviews the current evidence on effective stigma change strategies.

Scholars and scientists have pointed to persistent stigma as a major barrier to the success of mental health reform. Stigma occurs and so needs to be addressed at multiple levels of society including the structural level of institutional practices, laws, and regulations; among both the general public and groups, such as health care providers, employers, and landlords; and as self-stigma, which reflects internalized negative stereotypes.

The language that is used to discuss mental and substance use disorders, and to refer to people with these disorders, is often targeted for change as a strategy for reducing stigma. For example, many stakeholders prefer person-centered language, that is, language that describes a person as having a mental illness rather than as being mentally ill. The term "stigma" itself has been targeted for change by some stakeholder groups,

---

[1]For more information, see http://www.bazelon.org/ [October 2015].

and the Substance Abuse and Mental Health Services Administration (SAMHSA) is moving away from use of this term. In this report, the word stigma and its variants are used, except where the report discusses a more specific dimension of stigma such as prejudicial beliefs or discriminatory practices. We use patient-centered language throughout this report.

"Prejudice" means to prejudge and generally implies prejudgment based on erroneous beliefs or incomplete information. Similarly, stigma against people with mental or substance use disorders can stem from erroneous beliefs about, for example, their dangerousness or the unpredictability of their behavior. Lack of information about the nature of these disorders (e.g., their causes) can lead to public attitudes of shame and blame.

Discrimination is manifested as prejudice in behaviors that endorse differential treatment of people with mental and substance use disorders (Cummings et al., 2013). "Stereotyping" is the prejudicial characterization of an entire group, which blinds us to the differences among the people in that group. People with mental and substance use disorders are not a homogeneous group, and yet they are often referred to as such, for example, in discussions about background checks for firearm purchase.

The Americans with Disabilities Act (ADA) protects people with mental disorders against discrimination in many areas of civic life, and it defines discrimination to include a range of actions, for example, segregation of persons with mental disorders in public arenas, such as nursing homes and employment settings; screening that intends to or does screen out people with mental disorders; and failure to make reasonable accommodations to the known disability of an otherwise qualified individual with a mental illness. In 2003, the President's New Freedom Commission on Mental Health declared that recovery was possible and identified stigma and the fragmentation of the mental health care system among the major barriers to care. Subsequently, the ADA Amendments Act of 2008 (ADAAA) and other federal-level disability nondiscrimination laws expanded protections under the ADA, for example, by ensuring that a person with mental illness whose condition improved as a result of treatment continued to be protected under the law. Following the President's Commission and a 2006 SAMHSA Consensus Statement, we use "recovery" in this report to refer to an individually defined and nonlinear journey toward living a purposeful and satisfying life.

In addition to a fragmented mental health care system, the community of stakeholders concerned about mental and substance use disorders reflects a multiplicity of goals, and at times, different competing agendas. Stigma is a complex phenomenon that occurs at the structural level of policies and regulations (such as those covered by the ADA and ADAAA), at the general public level (including prejudicial attitudes and behaviors toward people with mental and substance use disorders), and at the level of self (in which the individual internalizes negative stereotypes).

To inform future anti-stigma efforts in the United States, this report describes the changes needed to improve the lives of people with mental and substance use disorders by reviewing the current evidence base for stigma change strategies at all levels and provides recommendations for future efforts.

BACKGROUND AND COMMITTEE CHARGE

Mental and substance use disorders are prevalent and among the most highly stigmatized health conditions in the United States. Worldwide, mental and substance use disorders are leading causes of morbidity and mortality. The social and disease burden of these disorders increased by 37 percent between 1990 and 2010, primarily due to demographic trends in population growth and aging (Whiteford et al., 2013).

In a national survey in 2014, 14 percent of U.S. adults said they had experienced a mental health problem within the past year; and 4 percent said that they had experienced a serious mental illness, one that met standard diagnostic criteria in the *Diagnostic and Statistical Manual of Mental Disorders* (Center for Behavioral Health Statistics and Quality, 2015).[2] In another survey regarding substance use, 24 million Americans aged 12 and older (9.4% of the population) said they had used illicit drugs in the past month, and 17 million (6.6%) reported alcohol dependence or misuse.[3] Of the nearly 23 million Americans who needed treatment (met standard criteria) for a drug or alcohol problem, less than one in ten received any treatment. Untreated substance use disorders reflect an estimated $417 billion in annual costs related to crime, health care services, and lost work productivity.[4] This estimate does not capture the many social costs of drug overdose and suicide.

A survey from SAMHSA (2014) provides detailed information on the use of health care services by people with mental disorders. People with a serious mental illness have a higher rate of service use than the general population of people with any mental illness (69% versus 45%) but treatment and services vary in quality and timeliness of delivery. Among adults who reported an unmet need for mental health care in the past year, the most common reasons were inability to afford the cost of care

---

[2] *Behavioral Health Trends in the United States: Results from the 2014 National Survey on Drug Use and Health.*

[3] Data from the National Institute on Drug Abuse. Available: htttps://www.drugabuse.gov/publications/drugfacts/nationwide-trends [April 2016].

[4] See https://www.drugabuse.gov/publications/drugfacts/nationwide-trends [April 2016].

(48%), believing that the problem could be handled without treatment (26.5%), not knowing where to go for services (25%), and not having the time to go for care (16%). Smaller proportions reported that they did not seek care because it might cause neighbors or the community to have a negative opinion (10%), they did not feel a need for treatment at the time (10%), they thought that treatment would not help (9%), they had fear of being committed to an institution or having to take medicine (9%), they had concerns about confidentiality and the potential negative effect on employment (8%), they did not want others to find out (6%), and they had no insurance coverage or inadequate coverage of mental health treatment (6% to 9%).

Mental illness and a history of substance misuse remain barriers to full participation in society in areas as basic as education, housing, and employment (Whitley and Henwood, 2014) and to fundamental rights of self-determination, such as access to the courts (Bazelon Center for Mental Health Law, 2014; Davis, 2010) and redress of grievances (Callard et al., 2012).

In the past, mental illness was considered a private matter rather than a public concern and a moral failing rather than a disease (Arboleda-Flórez and Stuart, 2012). Although stigma adheres to both mental illness and substance misuse, the degree of negative valuation varies across these disorders. In general, substance misuse is more highly stigmatized than mental illnesses and we have less evidence about what works to reduce it (Livingston et al., 2012). The public tends to hold people with addictions more responsible for their condition than they do people with a mental illness (Schomerus et al., 2011) and to report harsher reactions and greater unwillingness to socially include those with substance use disorders (Martin et al., 2000; McGinty et al., 2015).

Public attitudes about mental illness began to shift in the 1970s when media attention grew as a result of several factors including the availability of better treatments, a focus on the problem of "warehousing" people with mental illness in state institutions, and increased messaging to the public about mental illness and treatment. Deinstitutionalization policies brought people with mental illness out of state hospitals and into the public sphere, and the community, mental health movement arose with participation from former patients, their families, and treatment providers. Part of the overall deinstitutionalization plan had been to provide services at the local level, but community mental health services were underdeveloped and underfunded as the savings from closed hospitals was often redirected to cover state budget shortfalls (Grob, 1991). When the former residents of large, state-funded institutions returned to their communities, they often experienced poverty, homelessness, and discrimination. Mental health organizations launched public education campaigns to raise awareness about this crisis. With the increase in media coverage, people began to read about mental illness and the unmet needs of people with these disorders in the then-new health and science sections of their newspapers (Borinstein, 1992).

In 1950, the first major national study of public stigma was launched followed by three congressionally mandated studies in 1955, 1956, and 1976 (Pescosolido et al., 2000). These studies documented an extreme lack of public knowledge about the nature and causes of mental illness and a deep unwillingness to discuss mental illness. In 1989, the Robert Wood Johnson Foundation sponsored the first major study of Americans' attitudes toward mental health and illness. A review of public surveys since 1990 concluded that, although attitudes about mental illness have evolved, and there are marked differences across mental disorders, little is known about the relationship between attitudes and actual behaviors toward people with mental and substance use disorders (Angermeyer and Dietrich, 2006).

Combining data from these early studies with data from 1996, 2002, and 2006, researchers compared responses to analogous mental health and substance misuse modules in the General Social Survey. They found that public perceptions about the dangerousness and unpredictability of people with mental and substance use disorders have not decreased significantly over time. In fact, when asked to describe mental illness in 1996, a significantly larger proportion of the U.S. public spontaneously included a mention of violence than had done so in earlier surveys; and between 1991 and 2006, beliefs about the underlying cause of alcohol abuse shifted in the direction of moral blame (Pescosolido et al., 2010; Phelan et al., 2000; Schnittker, 2008).

Despite extensive research on stigma and general agreement that stigma is persistent, harmful, and discriminatory, the evidence about what works to change negative behavioral health social norms is sometimes conflicting and not uniformly robust (Livingston et al., 2012; Pescosolido, 2013; Stuart and Sartorius, 2005). There is less research on the subject of stigma against people with substance use disorders, but it is known that addiction stigma differs enough from mental illness stigma that lessons cannot always be transferred from one to the other (McGinty et al., 2015).

It is in this context that the Center for Behavioral Health Statistics and Quality at SAMHSA of the U.S. Department of Health and Human Services requested that the National Research Council and Institute of Medicine undertake a study of what is known about negative social norms and how to change them. In this report, the term "social norms" refers to a range of shared attitudes, beliefs, and behaviors directed toward people with mental and substance use disorders. Social norms are guides for behavior. Some norms are formalized as laws, such as those that prohibit issuance of a driver's license in some states to someone in a state psychiatric hospital, but many are informally understood and enforced through public sanctions, such as exclusion or reprimand. Erving Goffman's influential 1963 essay on stigma defines that term as a deeply discrediting attitude that reduces the bearer "from a whole and usual person to a tainted, discounted one" (Goffman, 1963). The next section provides an overview of stigma as it relates to mental illness and substance misuse. The full statement of task is in Box 1-1. This report focuses on the nature and dynamics of stigma and what the evidence shows about what has worked to change negative norms concerning mental and substance use disorders.

In addition to expertise in content areas, such as communications science and behavioral health, the committee included individuals with current experience or a history of mental or substance use disorders as individuals, family members, partners, caregivers, friends, and health care providers with experience of treating people with these disorders. Individuals with such knowledge and experience were sought and included through a nominations process that encouraged study sponsors and a wide range of other individuals and organizations to offer suggestions for committee membership. Once established, the committee also sought and included individuals with direct knowledge and experience of mental

---

BOX 1-1
Statement of Task

An ad hoc committee under the auspices of the National Research Council and the Institute of Medicine will examine the evidence base on strategies to change social norms, beliefs, and attitudes related to mental and substance use disorders. The U.S. Department of Health and Human Services' Center for Behavioral Health Statistics and Quality at the Substance Abuse and Mental Health Services Administration (SAMHSA) will use the recommendations for strategic planning within an ongoing program of research in the area of social norms and communications practices and to inform the SAMHSA Office of Communication's future activities to change behavioral health social norms.

The committee will review and discuss evidence on (1) the change in behavioral health norms needed to support individuals with mental and substance use disorders to seek treatment and other supportive services; (2) discrimination, negative attitudes, and stereotyping faced by individuals with mental health and/or substance use disorders; and (3) public knowledge about behavioral health, including how to seek help for people with such disorders.

The committee will issue a final report with recommendations to address the above issues.

and substance use disorders to participate in two public workshops that provided input to the committee, which contributed to the development of the report: see the workshop agendas in Appendix A.

OVERVIEW

Stigma can be defined as relationship between an attribute and a stereotype that assigns undesirable labels, qualities, and behaviors to a person. Labeled individuals are devalued socially, leading to inequality and discrimination (Link and Phelan, 2001). For example, when a person with schizophrenia (an attribute) is assumed to be violent (a stereotype), she or he will be considered dangerous (an undesirable label). This occurs despite data documenting that people with schizophrenia are more likely to be victims than perpetrators of violence (Teplin et al., 2005). There is debate at times about whether stigma actually arises from the label or from non-normative behavior on the part of the individual, but findings from public surveys in the United States indicate that, controlling for behavior, the label itself is stigmatizing (Pescosolido, 2013).

Discrimination against people with mental and substance use disorders deprives many individuals of opportunities in areas including education, housing, and competitive employment. Because the age of onset for some mental illnesses, including schizophrenia and bipolar disorder, is often the late teens and early twenties, stigma produces early life inequities at key transitional points of personal development and civic life (McLeod and Kaiser, 2004).

The literature on stigma characterizes three major interrelated types: structural, public, and self-stigma, along with courtesy stigma (directed toward family and friends of those with a mental or substance use disorder) and label avoidance. People avoid being labeled with a behavioral health problem because of concerns about resulting discrimination or social rejection, and although this certainly occurs, self-disclosure of mental or substance abuse disorders can also have positive outcomes related to help-seeking and feelings of inclusion. Label avoidance also negatively influences the decision to seek help for one's self or others (Corrigan, 2015).

For structural stigma, the committee adopted the definition put forward by Hatzenbuehler and Link (2014, p. 2): "societal-level conditions, cultural norms, and institutional practices that constrain the opportunities, resources, and wellbeing for stigmatized populations."

Public stigma describes negative attitudes, beliefs, and behaviors held within a community or the larger cultural context that are referred to collectively in this report as negative social norms. There may be intersecting stigmas, for example, of race or poverty and mental illness that increase the likelihood that a person will experience discrimination and injustice. Public stigma can predispose individuals in a community or other social group to fear, reject, avoid, and discriminate against people with mental illness (Parcesepe and Cabassa, 2013).

Self-stigma refers to the internalization of public stigma by a person with a mental or substance use disorder (Corrigan et al., 2014). This internalization can lead to denial of symptoms and rejection of treatment and contribute to the isolation of people with mental and substance use disorders from valuable social supports. Self-stigma does not emerge from lack of insight or intentional reaffirmation of negative social norms. It often arises as a result of previous experiences of discrimination or rejection. Self-stigma, like low self-efficacy, is a barrier along the path of recovery for people with mental and substance use disorders.

These discrete terms for the major levels and types of stigma reflect how the phenomenon has been defined by stakeholders, including researchers. Although there may be considerable overlap across the three types, the overall concept of stigma as a multilevel, multidimensional phenomenon facilitates research, measurement, and monitoring and can help to identify appropriate targets for change at each level. Researchers point to the presence of a "stigma complex," a system of interrelated, heterogeneous parts that operate in a dynamic process (Pescosolido, 2015).

Because stigma is fundamentally embedded and enacted in social relationships, as noted in the original classic treatise on stigma (Goffman, 1963), the phenomenon occurs at the intersection of individual and community factors. Initially, individual factors define the nature and extent of the "mark," which determines the probability of a label being given. This elicits the stigmatization process; however, cultural differences and the nature of the community shape the environment in which "difference" is defined, evaluated, and handled. For example, clear cross-national differences in mental illness stigma have been documented through analyses of newspapers across various countries (Olafsdottir and Beckfield, 2011) and related evidence linking prevalent public attitudes and the experiences of people with mental illness (Evans-Lacko et al., 2012a; Mojtabai, 2010).

Weaker stigmatizing responses are elicited when the stigmatized and the stigmatizer are more equal in social status and social power. As the power levels become more disparate, with the potential stigmatizer being more powerful, a stronger stigmatizing response will be elicited. For example, a strong stigmatizing response may include assigning a high level of severity to the condition, and thus the stigmatized individual will be subject to greater prejudice and discrimination. For example, in the context of health care, there can be a significant perceived or actual power differential between the provider and the patient. Stigma occurs in the health care system at both public and structural levels, that is, among health care provider groups and from the institution itself. This creates a feedback loop that engenders negative norms and increases self-stigma, which can negatively impact outcomes over the life course of stigmatized individuals (Gardner et al., 2011).

Effective stigma change initiatives attend to all relevant dimensions of the stigma complex, regardless of the specific level that is the target of the campaign. Both planned and unplanned impacts of campaign need to be considered in light of potential latent or unintended effects, for example, the potential negative effects of disclosing the experience of mental illness in a highly stigmatizing context. Conversely, there is evidence that addressing multiple levels of stigma within a campaign can create what Evans-Lacko calls a "virtuous cycle" to replace the harmful feedback loop among structural and public stigma and self-stigma (2012a).

BEHAVIORAL HEALTH IN THE U.S. CONTEXT

Throughout human history, conditions with no known cause or cure have been heavily freighted by stigma. As a dynamic, culture-bound phenomenon, stigma's severity and its impact on stigmatized individuals vary across time, place, and culture. There are many examples of stigmatizing conditions including cleft palate, epilepsy, HIV/AIDS, tuberculosis, and cancer, as well as mental and substance use disorders. Once causes and cures are developed, stigmas are often lessened (Grob, 1991).

At present, the lack of consensus in the United States about the origin, definition, and diagnosis of mental illnesses (Adam, 2013) may contribute to the maintenance of stigma. This is reflected by communities of stakeholders, which are divided across several domains. Although it is beyond the scope of this report to describe the perspectives and debates among the stakeholders, some current controversies that may impede efforts to combine and leverage resources to reduce stigma are briefly described in this section.

Different Diagnostics: DSM and RDoCs

The American Psychiatric Association's *Diagnostic and Statistical Manual of Mental Disorders* (DSM-5) places mental disorders in discrete categories on the basis of clinical signs and symptoms. These categories were established through the consensus of experts, and most recently updated amid controversy in 2013 (Frances and Widiger, 2012). Other experts in the field prefer to move away from discrete categories toward the concept of dimensionality in which mental illnesses overlap, and to base the diagnostic system for mental illness on research data rather than symptom-based categories (Cuthbert, 2014).

Other recent changes include new emphasis on the importance of strengths-based approaches to assessment and treatment of mental disorders, which has been championed by consumer and advocacy groups (Xie, 2013), and increased attention to the role of childhood trauma and exposure to historical and cultural violence, through trauma-informed care and the use of screening tools including the Adverse Childhood Experience Scale. Other new approaches to psychiatric assessment include social and environmental factors that influence the development and trajectory of mental and substance use disorders (see, e.g., Chisolm and Lyketsos, 2012).

To address these concerns, in 2010, the National Institutes of Mental Health (NIMH) launched the Research Domain Criteria (RDoC) project. RDoC supports research that is focused on dimensional variables, such as motivation and reward, or brain circuits that are dysregulated in many mental illnesses (Adam, 2013). But there have also been criticisms of the RDoC project. One is that it is a type of scientific reductionism, which was successful in understanding and developing treatments for physical illnesses, but may not adequately address the heterogeneous nature of psychopathology or the complexities of human consciousness and subjective experience that underlie mental and substance use disorders (Parnas, 2014). Taking the two approaches together, DSM-5 provides a clinical tool for diagnosis of mental illness, and a set of reimbursable categories for payment and coverage, whereas the NIMH-supported brain research community will shed light on the neurobiological underpinnings of psychopathology to inform future editions of DSM (Adam, 2013; Maj, 2014).

Different Agendas: Rights and Services

There are two quite different perspectives concerning the best or most useful approach to helping people with mental illness or substance use disorders—one of services and one of rights. A services agenda has the goal of increasing access to and quality of health care services by people with mental and substance use disorders; a rights agenda applies a social justice approach to eliminate discrimination and promote equality and full civil rights (Corrigan, 2015). The rights agenda is grassroots in nature and has the support of many people with firsthand experience of stigma and discrimination. Consumer and advocacy groups have stressed the importance of self-efficacy (empowerment) and access to opportunities for personal and social advancement in recovery. As noted above, stigma can negatively impact self-efficacy, help-seeking, and social inclusion (Ostrow and Adams, 2012).

Services agendas are underpinned by research showing that a significant proportion of people with mental illness do not seek treatment (Wang et al., 2002). This is due, in part, to public and structural stigma (Clement et al., 2015) as well as self-stigma, and label avoidance (Corrigan, 2015). A concern on the part of some behavioral health experts is that services agendas and mental health services researchers do not focus on people who are not seeking treatment and that this is a population in need of research attention. Understanding how these agendas both align and compete with each other is a critical step in setting national goals for stigma reduction.

Different Models: Medical and Recovery

Many health care professionals continue to be skeptical about the possibility of recovery from some mental and substance use disorders despite evidence to the contrary (Harding et al., 1987a, 1987b). Although treatment is thought to be beneficial on the whole, in one survey, one-half of the respondents who were health professionals did not endorse recovery as an outcome for serious mental illness (Magliano et al., 2004). This view derives at least in part from a biomedical model of mental illness, which looks for causes of psychiatric symptoms in the neurobiology and neurophysiology of the brain. Health professionals' skepticism about the possibility of recovery as "cure" has been shown to increase public stigma (Henderson et al., 2014; Schomerus et al., 2012) and to contribute to negative public attitudes about the potential for recovery (Henderson et al., 2014). The analogous brain disease model of addiction also has both critics and supporters. The hope of the research community is that efforts to understand the neurobiological underpinnings of addiction may contribute to the development of effective treatment and prevention strategies (Volkow and Koob, 2015).

Although the concept of recovery from mental illness has a long history, the modern mental health recovery movement in the United States has its roots in the Civil Rights era of the 1960s and the consumer movements of the 1980s and 1990s, including the consumer, survivor, and ex-patient movements, which gained early support from SAMHSA. Underpinning these efforts was the evidence from research conducted by Harding and colleagues on recovery from mental illness (Harding et al., 1987a, 1987b). These efforts along with the deinstitutionalization policies of the 1970s also spurred the development of peer-services movements of the 1980s and 1990s (Anthony, 2000). More recently, the 1999 Surgeon General's Report and the 2003 President's New Freedom Commission on Mental Health encouraged a national paradigm shift toward the mental health recovery model.

Recovery in the context of substance use disorders has roots in the Anonymous movement, beginning, for example, with Alcoholics Anonymous (AA), which began in the 1930s, and Narcotics Anonymous (NA), which was joined with AA but later established as separate organization. The concept of recovery regarding substance use disorders overlaps but also differs from that of mental illness, notably in the degree to which recovery is thought to include responsibility to society and peers. For AA and NA members, giving back to the community as peers is the 12th and last step to recovery. Although these various peer and consumer movements may vary in terms of priorities and goals, they largely agree on the importance of empowerment and equality for people with or labeled with mental and substance use disorders (Ostrow and Adams, 2012).

THE BROADER U.S. CONTEXT

The Health Care System

Although stigma may contribute to the low quality of mental illness and addiction services in the United States (Schulze, 2007; Schulze and Angermeyer, 2003), several features of the nation's health care system also contribute to the current situation. They include the fragmented bureaucracy for accessing behavioral health care (Garfield, 2011); overuse of coercive approaches to care; rejection of facilities by communities; and lower funding for research in the areas of behavioral health treatment and services than for neuroscience and physical health treatment and services (Heflinger and Hinshaw, 2010; Schomerus and Angermeyer, 2008; Schulze, 2007; Schulze and Angermeyer, 2003).

Most behavioral health services in the United States are financed through public sources. For mental health services, Medicaid programs are the principle payers. Treatment for alcohol and drug use disorders is funded largely by state and local non-Medicaid sources. Care utilization types and rates vary widely by age, sex, insurance status, and severity of illness. For example, children are most likely to receive behavioral health care from specialty providers or the education system. Among adults, women are more likely to obtain services from the general medical sector, while men are more likely to obtain services from specialty providers. The complexity of behavioral health care funding and service delivery systems challenges policy makers' efforts to implement and evaluate programs as part of health care reform (Garfield, 2011).

Current efforts toward the integration of behavioral health and primary (and other physical) care in the nation's health care system offer possibilities for breaking down the walls that separate physical health from mental health both in treatment and in the educational preparation of health care professionals (Mechanic et al., 2013). One bias against people with mental illness in the health care system is a form of stigmatization that results in misattribution of physical symptoms of illness to concurrent mental disorders (Pescosolido et al., 2008a; Sartorius et al., 2010; Thornicroft et al., 2007). In addition, primary care practitioners are less likely to refer patients with mental illnesses to appropriate physical health services, such as mammography, cardiovascular procedures, and pain management (Corrigan and Kleinlein, 2005; Druss et al., 2000). Access to lifesaving medical technologies, such as cardiac catheterization and revascularization procedures, is also less likely for people with mental disorders due to socioeconomic factors, lack of insurance, geographic remoteness from tertiary medical centers, and cognitive impairment that complicates informed consent and effective provision of aftercare (Druss et al., 2000). People with serious mental illness die at younger ages than the general population. Research that analyzed data from the public mental health system across the United States showed that, in comparison with the general population, individuals in this population lose decades of potential life that vary by state and year from 13 to 30 years (Colton and Manderscheid, 2006).

Social Justice and Inequality

Mental Illness and Incarceration

In the United States, the mental health system and the criminal justice system are unfortunately closely linked. More than one-half of all inmates in the United States have a mental health problem (James and Glaze, 2006). Mental illness, drug addiction, neighborhood poverty, and school dropouts are factors that increase the risk of involvement with the criminal justice system. Blacks and Hispanics are disproportionately affected by disparities in the system, from arrest through parole release, which have a substantial cumulative effect on their rates of incarceration (National Research Council, 2014a). As a result in part of mandatory drug sentencing, women have had the fastest growing incarceration rate in the United States since the 1970s (The Sentencing Project, 2012),[5] and women are more likely than men to enter prison with an existing mental illness (James and Glaze, 2006). Socioeconomic disadvantage subsequently hampers the successful reentry in society of released offenders and increases the risk of reincarceration. Prisons also lack resources for the diagnosis and treatment of inmates with existing mental health conditions, and prison conditions, most notably overcrowding and solitary confinement,

---

[5]Women are more likely to be in prison for drug and property offenses, whereas men are more likely to be in prison for violent offenses.

can contribute to the development of mental illness in people who previously did not have them. (National Research Council, 2014a).

Young People and the Criminal Justice System

Young people are at particular risk for involvement with the criminal justice system. Adolescent behavior is driven by age-related developmental risk factors that bring them to the attention of the justice system, such as novelty-seeking and interest in experimentation, sensitivity to external influences (peer pressure), and lack of capacity for self-regulation. "Get-tough" policies of previous decades criminalized millions of young people for illegal behaviors that most would have abandoned as they developed cognitively and matured socially. Policies that lowered the maximum age of juvenile court assignment and excluded certain violent crimes from juvenile jurisdiction placed young people in the adult courts.

Improvements in various states and jurisdictions have been implemented in recent years, including raising the age at which juvenile court jurisdiction ends, but reform of the justice system will also require a developmental approach to juvenile justice based on evidence concerning adolescent growth and development and effective age-relevant interventions (National Research Council, 2014b). At the present time, the criminal justice system does not consistently provide young people with the social conditions they need to develop into emotionally self-regulated, healthy, and productive adults (National Research Council, 2014a). This places youths at risk for developing mental and substance use disorders, even when they do not have these disorders at the time of arrest and incarceration, and negatively influences the life trajectories of incarcerated youths, especially among racial and ethnic minority groups (National Research Council, 2014a).

Structural Discrimination

Legislation concerning people with mental illness tends to use broad, homogeneous inclusion criteria (people with any diagnosis of mental illness) rather than more specific and objective measures of cognitive or functional impairment or reduced capacity (Corrigan et al., 2005b). Arbitrariness is a defining feature of structural stigma, reflecting the stereotype that all people with mental illness are dangerous or inadequate in some way, and therefore "deserve" restricted liberties and reduced opportunities. In fact, people with mental and substance use disorders are not a discrete, static, or homogeneous group. There is considerable variability across behavioral health conditions; among individuals in the severity, symptomatology, and expression of these conditions; and across the lifespan of each person with a mental or substance use disorder.

Lack of parity for mental health coverage was among the most significant forms of structural discrimination in the United States that ended with the passage of the Mental Health Parity and Addiction Equity Act in 2008 after a multidecade fight. Paired with the Affordable Care Act, which prevents insurance companies from denying coverage to people with pre-existing conditions, including schizophrenia, depression, bipolar disorder, and drug or alcohol disorders, and allows people to remain on their parent's health plans until the age of 26, these legislative changes represent major steps forward in advancing the rights of people with mental and substance use disorders.

Unfortunately, other forms of structural discrimination persist despite protections offered by the ADA and the ADAAA of 2008, which expanded protections for people with mental illness, along with the Fair Housing Act (Bazelon Center for Mental Health Law, 2014; Stuart, 2006). Inadequate enforcement of legislation may be a factor in the poorer outcomes observed for people with mental illness across legal, educational, employment, housing, and health care spheres.

THE COMMITTEE'S WORK AND THE REPORT

Input from the Field

In addition to analysis of the peer-reviewed literature, the committee held two public workshops to obtain input from a wide variety of stakeholders in the many domains reflected in its statement of task (see Box 1-1 above). The first workshop was designed to identify lessons learned from efforts to change negative social norms in health-related areas outside of behavioral health. The second workshop was designed to focus on the application of these lessons to mental health and substance use disorder issues in the United States. At the workshops, experts offered perspectives on anti-stigma efforts related to epilepsy, tobacco use, HIV/AIDS, and lung cancer, in addition to mental and substance use disorders.

Principles Guiding the Study

The committee operationalized its task to focus on the current understanding of stigma and its effect on the lives of people with mental and substance use disorders and their families and friends, evidence concerning the success and failure of both domestic efforts to reduce stigma and similar efforts in other countries, and the research needed to inform and evaluate future efforts in the United States. More specifically, to develop the report and its recommendations, the committee focused on four basic questions:

1. What works to reduce stigma against people with mental illness and substance use disorders?
2. For whom (for which target groups) does it work?
3. Under which circumstances does it work? Or, what characterizes successful efforts?
4. How does one know it worked? What is the evidence?

In the conduct of this study, the committee held both closed and open sessions, as well as the two workshops, and commissioned eight background papers to address a wide range of research questions. Discussions in the open sessions and during the workshops were intended to be inclusive of a broad range of viewpoints, and the committee heard divergent opinions on many topics, including the connotation of several relevant terms, especially the term stigma. Some people expressed concern that the use of the word stigma may itself have a stigmatizing effect, or that it underemphasizes the unequal treatment and discrimination faced by people with mental illness that is referred to in this report as structural stigma, but there is no consensus among stakeholders on the deleterious influence of the term stigma (Corrigan, 2014; Corrigan and Ben Zeev, 2012). In this report, the word stigma is used to refer to a range of negative attitudes, beliefs, and behaviors about mental illness and substance use disorders. A more specific term, such as negative beliefs, is used to express a particular concept, for example, disbelief in the efficacy of medications in treating mental illnesses, or in the possibility of recovery.

Structure of the Report

Chapter 2 provides a summary of current understanding of attitudes, beliefs, and behavioral dispositions toward people with mental and substance use disorders and identifies the major gaps in the scientific knowledge base on stigma.

Chapter 3 describes a communications science framework that should form the basis of a stigma change campaign. The chapter describes effective means for reaching target audiences, choosing message sources and media for delivery, and designing messages that achieve the goals and objectives of a campaign.

Chapter 4 presents the evidence on the effectiveness of stigma change strategies, including legislative and policy interventions, education, interventions that promote positive social contact between people with and without behavioral disorders (contact-based programs), advocacy, and protest. The committee summarizes the findings from three national-level stigma change campaigns from Australia, Canada, and England that represent a relevant evidence base.

Chapter 5 outlines a research strategy for planning, implementation, and evaluation of stigma change campaigns, including a discussion of measurement of stigma-related constructs, research and design considerations, and cost-benefit analyses. The committee suggests areas of research and research questions for future inquiry into the nature of stigma and stigma change.

Chapter 6 applies lessons learned from previous stigma change efforts in the context of U.S. health care, social, and legal systems. The chapter provides the committee's conclusions and recommendations concerning communications science; peer services, and other contact-based programs; public and structural anti-stigma campaigns; and the components of an effective national-level strategy to eliminate prejudice and discrimination against people with mental and substance use disorders.

2

Understanding Stigma of Mental and Substance Use Disorders

The term "stigma" is used throughout this chapter and the report to represent the complex of attitudes, beliefs, behaviors, and structures that interact at different levels of society (i.e., individuals, groups, organizations, systems) and manifest in prejudicial attitudes about and discriminatory practices against people with mental and substance use disorders. Attention to stigmatizing structures of society, such as laws and regulations, enables examination of prejudice and discrimination against people with mental and substance use disorders. Discriminatory policies and practices can appear to endorse negative social norms and deepen self-stigma.

This chapter offers a brief overview of what is currently understood about stigma, including influencing factors and consequences of stigma from the level of society as a whole to the experience of people with behavioral health disorders. Targets for change and interventions for changing stigmatizing attitudes, beliefs, and behaviors are discussed in Chapter 4.

FINDINGS FROM SURVEYS OF PUBLIC KNOWLEDGE AND NORMS

Public knowledge and norms about people with mental and substance use disorders have been captured through population-based surveys with components focused on the stigma of mental and substance use disorders as it is reflected in stereotypes, help- or treatment-seeking, and behavioral dispositions.

Results of an analysis of the National Comorbidity Survey-Replication that compared data from the early 1990s and early 2000s showed that stigma associated with mental health treatment decreased, and support among the general public for treatment-seeking increased (Mojtabai, 2007). A survey of states in 2007 and 2009 showed that more than 80 percent of U.S. adults agreed that mental illness treatment is effective; people living in states with higher per capita expenditures on mental health services were more likely to agree that treatment is effective and were more likely to report receiving treatment (Centers for Disease Control and Prevention et al., 2012).

The Substance Abuse and Mental Health Services Administration (2014), as detailed in Chapter 1, found that some common reasons reported for not receiving behavioral health care included inability to afford the cost of care (48%), believing that the problems could be handled without treatment (26.5%), not knowing where to go for services (25%), concerns about confidentiality (10%), that it might cause neighbors or the community to have a negative opinion (10%), that it might cause a negative effect on a person's job (8%), fear of being committed (10%), inadequate or no coverage of mental health treatment (6% to 9%), and thinking that treatment would not help (9%).

Comparing results of the 1996 General Social Survey (GSS) stigma modules with those of surveys in the 1950s on U.S. attitudes about mental illness stigma showed that public knowledge about mental and substance use disorders increased, specifically as it related to the neurobiological underpinnings of these disorders. There was greater public awareness of the stigma associated with these disorders, but public stigma itself remained high (Pescosolido, 2013; Pescosolido et al., 2010). Results from the 2006 GSS found greater sophistication in the public's knowledge of disorders and treatment than in the 1996 survey administration, but stigma levels for people with mental illness did not decrease over time (Pescosolido et al., 2010).

Results of the GSS have also shown that the level of public stigma varies along a gradient of social distance. In more intimate settings, the rate of stigma reflected as social rejection was higher, for example, a depressed person to "marry into the family" (60.5% rejection rate) versus the more distant "move next door" (22.9% rejection rate). Stigma against children and adolescents was lower compared to that of adults and also varied with social distance reporting higher rates of rejection for a friend with depression (29%) than for a classmate with depression (11%). One-half of all adult respondents said that treatment would result in discrimination and long-term negative effects on a child's future (Pescosolido, 2013)

Across countries surveyed in the Stigma in Global Context Study, levels of recognition, acceptance of neurobiological causes of mental illness and substance use, and treatment endorsement were similarly high; however, a core of five prejudice items persisted. The researchers called this the "backbone of stigma": issues of trust in intimate settings such as the family, potential contact with a vulnerable group such as children, the potential for self-harm, mental illness being antithetical to power or authority, and uneasiness about how to interact with people with mental illness (Pescosolido et al., 2013).

Finally, a review of studies of public stigma of mental illness, which included studies with variables related to substance use disorders, showed that over time the proportion of Americans who endorse neuroscientific views of schizophrenia and alcohol dependence has grown (Pescosolido, 2013). Americans also have endorsed the use of physicians and prescription medication for these disorders in greater numbers and reported being more willing to discuss behavioral health difficulties with family and friends. However, the persistence of core prejudice factors help explain why increased public knowledge has not decreased public stigma. Core indicators of stigma remain higher for people with schizophrenia and substance disorders than other conditions. Further, the highly stigmatizing public perception of violence as a component of mental illness has not decreased over time.

FACTORS THAT INFLUENCE STIGMA

In this chapter and throughout the report, in discussing stigma we begin with structural stigma and work from it to public stigma and self-stigma. This ordering reflects the committee's views on the relationships among the three levels of stigma and on the importance of addressing structural stigma and its consequences as a means for also reducing public and self-stigma. Societal structures reflect public norms and values, and many of the factors that influence structural stigma are the same as those that influence public stigma. Self-stigma occurs when a person with mental or substance use disorder internalizes negative stereotypes and the public and structural stigma directed at these disorders.

Public perceptions and beliefs about mental and substance use disorders are influenced by knowledge about these disorders, the degree of contact or experience that one has had with people with mental and substance use disorders, and media portrayal of people with mental and substance use disorders, as well as media coverage of tragic events, notably gun violence and suicide (Swanson et al., 2015). Public perceptions are also strongly influenced by social norms concerning the attribution of cause, or blame, for mental and substance use disorders, and the perceived dangerousness or unpredictability of people with these disorders. Race, ethnicity, and culture are embedded in social relationships and as such play a role in shaping attitudes, beliefs, and behaviors.

Blame

A biogenic model of the origins of mental and substance use disorders has been applied in an effort to reduce blame and promote positive attitudes about the value of treatment and the possibility of recovery. People with substance use disorders are generally considered to be more responsible for their conditions than people with depression, schizophrenia, or other psychiatric disorders (Crisp et al., 2000, 2005; Lloyd, 2013; Schomerus et al., 2011). Belief that a substance misuser's illness is a result of the person's own behavior can also influence attitudes about the value and appropriateness of publicly funded alcohol and drug treatment and services (Olsen et al., 2003).

There is a lack of empirical evidence supporting the stigma-reducing benefits of a neurobiological conceptualization of psychiatric illness (Trujols, 2015). Although some research suggests that attributing mental illness to biological causes may reduce the blame placed on individuals for their behavior (Rosenfield, 1997), other research has shown that attributing behavior to a genetic cause can increase perceptions of the difference of people with the disorder, and of the persistence, seriousness, and possible transmissibility of mental illness (Phelan, 2005). Overall, promulgation of the brain disease model of addiction does not appear to have reduced public stigma about substance use disorders and may decrease perceptions of self-efficacy and ability to cope among people with behavioral health disorders (Trujols, 2015).

Stereotypes of Dangerousness and Unpredictability

Americans are more likely to believe in the dangerousness of people with mental illness than are citizens of other developed, industrialized nations (Jorm and Reavley, 2014). In a recent national survey, four in ten Americans believed that children and adolescents with depression were likely to be violent, a finding that may be related to media coverage of school shooting incidents (Pescosolido, 2013). Stereotypes of violence and unpredictability are associated with higher levels of public stigma toward people with mental illness (Martin et al., 2000, 2007; Perry, 2011; Phelan et al., 2000). People with substance use disorders are considered even more dangerous and unpredictable than those with schizophrenia or depression (Schomerus et al., 2011). In a survey conducted in the United States (Link et al., 1997), a vast majority of respondents considered it likely for a cocaine- or alcohol-dependent person to hurt others. People are less likely to endorse the stereotype of violence if they have had direct contact with people who have mental and substance use disorders and have not experienced violent acts by people with these disorders (Jorm and Reavley, 2014).

Stereotypes of dangerousness can influence public policy in terms of restricting the rights of persons with behavioral disorders (Pescosolido et al., 1999). In the current context of the increasing frequency of mass shootings in the United States (Blair and Schweit, 2013), beliefs about the dangerousness of persons with mental illness and substance use disorders have come to the forefront in public policy debates. To inform these debates, a review of epidemiological findings related to mental illness, gun violence, and suicide found that there is a greater relative risk of violence in people with mental illness than those without mental illness, but the risk is actually very small. The risk of violence is greater for people with schizophrenia, bipolar disorder, co-occurring substance use disorder, and those exposed to certain socioeconomic factors, such as poverty, crime victimization, early life trauma, and a high neighborhood crime rate (Swanson et al., 2015). People with substance use disorders and antisocial personality disorders have a higher risk of violence than people with other psychiatric disorders (Fazel et al., 2009). The risk of suicide, as another form of violence, is increased by concurrent substance use; symptoms, such as hopelessness and depression; psychotic disorders; bipolar disorder; and environmental factors, such as access to guns and media reporting of suicide (Swanson et al., 2015). Swanson and colleagues point to the gaps in the knowledge base on the relationship between behavioral disorders, violence, suicide, and guns, as well as to the gaps in knowledge on effective policies to reduce gun violence and suicide.

Knowledge about Mental and Substance Use Disorders

Knowledge about mental and substance use disorders can positively influence public norms, yet there is evidence that reframing these disorders as brain diseases produces mixed results on people's attitudes and behavior toward people with mental and substance disorders. As noted above, public education campaigns that frame mental and substance use disorders as brain diseases can have unintended consequences, including increased perception of difference and disbelief in the likelihood of recovery (Pescosolido et al., 2010; Schomerus et al., 2012; Trujols, 2015).

People with substance use disorders, in particular, are viewed by the public as weak-willed (Schomerus et al., 2011) although evidence shows that they are as likely to adhere to treatment as people with other chronic medical conditions, such as hypertension or diabetes (McLellan et al., 2000). Unfortunately, and in spite of efforts to educate the public, this misperception has increased over time according to the findings from national surveys in 1996 and 2006 (Pescosolido et al., 2010). Media portrayals of people with untreated and symptomatic substance use disorders, rather than depictions of those on a path to recovery, may be a factor in maintaining or increasing negative stereotypes and stigmatizing attitudes and beliefs about people with substance use disorders (McGinty et al., 2015).

Among health care providers, one consequence of bias against mental illness is the misattribution of physical symptoms of illness to concurrent mental disorders (Pescosolido et al., 2008b; Sartorius et al., 2010; Thornicroft et al., 2007), as well as lower rates of referral by primary care practitioners to appropriate physical health services like mammography, cardiovascular procedures, and pain management (Corrigan and Kleinlein, 2005).

Health care practitioners outside fields of behavioral health also lack knowledge about mental illness, and there is evidence that this can lead to misdiagnosis of both mental and physical conditions, and to selection of improper and inadequate treatment regimens (Wang et al., 2002). In addition to knowledge gaps, negative attitudes toward individuals who have mental or substance use disorders are prevalent among health care providers (Meltzer et al., 2013; Van Boekel et al., 2013). For example, although high remission rates for alcohol dependence have been found in population-based studies (Bischof et al., 2005), many health professionals continue to view alcoholism as incurable. In one study, nurses' self-reported lack of knowledge related to behavioral health was associated with greater reported fear and avoidance of people with mental illness (Ross and Goldner, 2009), demonstrating the link between lack of knowledge and the holding of prejudicial beliefs. Conversely, emergency room staff who reported having skills in treating these disorders held more positive views about the possibility of recovery than those who did not report having these skills (Clarke et al., 2014).

Contact and Experience

People's immediate social networks and the extent of their contact with people with mental illness affect their understanding of and opinions about mental illness in general (Chandra and Minkovitz, 2006; Corrigan and Penn, 1999). However, increased contact with people with mental illness does not necessarily reduce stigmatizing beliefs, and some studies have found that contact with people with substance use disorders raises the level of stigma (Lloyd, 2013). Among health professionals, negative attitudes toward people with substance use disorders increased over time during which they would have had more contact with people with those disorders (Christison and Haviland, 2003; Geller et al., 1989; Lindberg et al., 2006).

Several factors may explain why contact with people with mental and substance use disorders sometimes deepens stigma, including the affected individuals' symptom severity and stage of recovery; and, in the context of contact-based interventions, the quality of the intervention itself, the fidelity with which it was implemented, and the quality of the peer training that had been provided to the individuals offering the contact services. (Peer support services are discussed in greater detail in Chapter 4).

Medical students in Australia reported more positive attitudes about illicit drug users after they experienced contact with them in small-group settings (Silins et al., 2007). In a qualitative study of pharmacists and drug users in a needle exchange program in the United Kingdom, both groups reported a decreased sense of stigma with increasing contact and familiarity (Lloyd, 2013). A review of two similar studies found that college students for whom at least 50 percent of their friends used drugs scored lower on a measure of public stigma (Adlaf et al., 2009). In another study, people who had a family member with an alcohol use disorder reported lower levels of stigma toward alcohol users than those without a diagnosed family member (Kulesza et al., 2013). A lower level of stigma does not imply support for substance misuse; rather, it reflects more positive attitudes toward people with substance use disorders.

Importantly, despite these variations in outcomes, the bulk of available evidence suggests that there is a strong and consistent inverse relationship between contact as an intervention and the level of stigma; more contact with people with mental and substance use disorders is associated with lower levels of stigma related to these disorders. (This topic is discussed in the review of stigma change interventions in Chapter 4).

Media Portrayals

The media provide ideas about and images of behavioral health that influence public attitudes, beliefs, and behaviors toward people with mental and substance use disorders (Edney, 2004; Klin and Lemish, 2008; Nairn et al, 2011; Nawková et al., 2012). An example of the role of media comes from a study of mainstream publications from 1998 to 2008 that covered the topic of postpartum depression and other mental illnesses. The test of communication theories showed that the media's portrayals helped shape the public's opinions about postpartum depression and that when the attention given to postpartum depression and other types of mental illness was negative, public opinion tended to mirror negative perceptions (Holman, 2011).

Much of the evidence on the media's influence on stigma change is negative in direction (Pugh et al., 2015). The media play a crucial role in stoking fear and intensifying the perceived dangers of persons with substance use disorders (Lloyd, 2013). Similarly, media portrayals of people with mental illness are often violent, which promotes associations of mental illness with dangerousness and crime (Diefenbach and West, 2007; Klin and Lemish, 2008; Wahl et al., 2002). Furthermore, the media often depict treatment as unhelpful (Sartorius et al., 2010; Schulze, 2007) and portray pessimistic views of illness management and the possibility of recovery (Schulze, 2007).

There has been some positive change. An analysis of newspaper articles between 1989 and 1999 (Wahl et al., 2002) showed more coverage of issues related to stigma and mental health insurance parity in 1999 than 1989. The analysis also found that there were fewer articles that contained themes of dangerousness and negative tones in 1999 than in 1989. However, even in 1999, articles with themes of danger and negative tones were still more prevalent than positive themes in reported stories that included a focus on mental illness.

Another content analysis of a nationally representative sample of U.S. news coverage of mental health issues found that, in 39 percent of stories, an association was made between persons with mental illness and dangerousness (Corrigan et al., 2005a). Treatment was discussed in 26 percent of stories but only 16 percent of the stories included recovery as an outcome. Moreover, recent research suggests that, given the broad reach of U.S. media, the volume and intensity of negative coverage about mental and substance use disorders are increasing mental health stigma in other countries as well (Jorm and Reavley, 2014).

Studies of new social media, experimental studies, and evaluations of anti-stigma initiatives point to the potential value and capacity of the media to counter stigma. For example, in a study of tweets comparing the use of words that referred to schizophrenia and diabetes (Joseph et al., 2015), researchers found that tweets about schizophrenia were more likely to be negative, medically inappropriate, and sarcastic than tweets about diabetes. But their results also suggested that such public misinformation could also be a target for anti-stigma efforts targeted at young people.

Media reporting of suicide can be stigmatizing through selective reporting on homicides and suicides, especially celebrity suicides, but they can also be platforms for prevention by providing positive messaging about available support and resources, coping, mastering personal crises, and the value of help-seeking (Niederkrotenthaler et al., 2014). One study of social media reactions to an attempted suicide showed that a greater proportion of microblogs expressed caring, empathy, or calling for help (37%) than posts that were cynical or indifferent (23%) (Fu et al.,

2015). More research is needed to identify effective strategies that combine media, education, and support for help-seeking (Niederkrotenthaler et al., 2014).

In an experimental study that compared attitudinal outcomes, researchers found that stories of recovery decreased prejudiced attitudes toward people with mental illness and drug addiction and increased belief in treatment efficacy (McGinty et al., 2015). Australia's beyondblue campaign, a comprehensive social marketing campaign to destigmatize depression, provides another example of the impact of positive portrayals of mental illness. The researchers assessed changes in attitudes among the general public, controlling for different levels of exposure to the campaign, and found an increase in understanding of depression, awareness of discrimination, and self-reported use of mental health treatment (Jorm et al., 2005, 2006). (The beyondblue campaign, along with other national-scale stigma change efforts is discussed, in greater detail in Chapter 4.)

Race, Ethnicity, and Culture

Sociodemographic characteristics have been found to affect a large number of social beliefs, but when applied to stigma, the research findings are unclear (Pescosolido, 2013). Also important, the effect of sociodemographic characteristics differs depending on whether one is looking at the stigmatizer or the stigmatized person (Manago, 2015). Research is clearer on the relationship between culture, race, and ethnicity, and the quality of care that people receive (Bink, 2015). Ethnic and racial minorities access mental health care at a lower rate than whites, and when they do, the care they receive is often suboptimal (Schraufnagel et al., 2006; Substance Abuse and Mental Health Services Administration, 1999).

Several factors influence access, quality of care, and rates of treatment for mental disorders among ethnic and racial minorities and immigrant groups (Giacco et al., 2014; Schraufnagel et al., 2006). Quality of care is compromised by language barriers and provider misunderstanding of cultural ideas about illness, health, and treatment. Although most health care professionals agree that cultural competency training is important, lack of cultural awareness remains a problem in many health care settings (Giacco et al., 2014). Provision of physical and behavioral health services in integrated care settings has been shown to increase participation in mental health treatment for racial and ethnic minorities (Giacco et al., 2014; Schraufnagel et al., 2006).

CONSEQUENCES OF STIGMA

As defined in Chapter 1 and discussed in the introduction to this chapter, there are three distinct types of stigma: structural, public, and self. Figure 2-1 depicts these three main types of stigma and the consequences that result from each, as well as the possible targets for change and interventions that have been used to change stigmatizing attitudes, beliefs, and behaviors. This section reviews the evidence on the consequences of each type of stigma on both adults and children. However, because of the negative impacts of stigma on children and adolescents, we provide a separate discussion about young people with behavioral disorders from the perspective of the public, youth, families, and professionals.

Structural Stigma

Research on structural stigma is still in a developmental phase, and the research that has been done focuses primarily on mental illness rather than substance use disorders. While there is overlap between structural and public stigma, it is possible to define and distinguish between these phenomena. As shown in Figure 2-1, structural stigma is the societal and institutional manifestation of the attitudes, beliefs, and behaviors that create and perpetuate prejudice and discrimination. This section discusses structural stigma using examples of persistent prejudice and discrimination in public and private institutions, including government and legal systems, legislative bodies, employers, and educational institutions; health care and treatment systems; and the criminal justice system, including law enforcement, correctional institutions, and the courts.

Public and Private Institutions

One approach to operationalizing measurements of structural stigma has been through review of policies explicitly targeted at people with mental illness. A review of legislation in all 50 states found legal restrictions for people with mental illness in the following five domains: serving on a jury, voting, holding political office, parental custody rights, and marriage (Burton, 1990; Hemmens et al., 2002). A similar review of nearly 1,000 mental health-related proposed bills in 2002 found that 3 percent restricted liberties (e.g., allowed compulsory community treatment); 1 percent were discriminatory (e.g., restrictions on gun ownership, parental rights, placement of mental health facilities); and 4 percent reduced privacy (e.g., permitting disclosure of mental health information in special circumstances) (Corrigan et al., 2005b).

Although the National Alliance on Mental Illness (NAMI) described

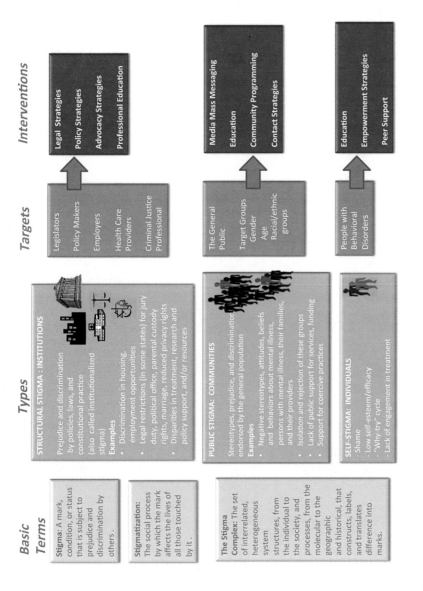

FIGURE 2-1 Stigma types, consequences, targets, and interventions.

many states' mental health systems as being in disrepair, their report on state legislation in 2014 documented increased activity on mental health issues. For example, in seven states, legislation was enacted to protect the rights of individuals who are civilly committed, to clarify and improve civil commitment proceedings, and to encourage community-based court ordered treatment (National Alliance on Mental Illness, 2014).

Ironically, although much attention focuses on the dangerousness and violence of people with mental illness, numerous studies have found that they are at higher risk of victimization (Choe et al., 2008; Desmarais et al., 2014; Khalifeh et al., 2015; Wolff et al., 2007) and of experiencing unfair treatment by authorities when they attempt to report crimes than people without mental illness (Pettitt et al., 2013). Poorer legal outcomes are also observed among plaintiffs with mental illness in employment discrimination suits in comparison with plaintiffs without mental illness (Swanson et al., 2006).

People with mental illness are more likely to experience housing and employment discrimination and homelessness than people without mental illness (Corbière et al., 2011; Corrigan and Shapiro, 2010; Corrigan et al., 2006b). Two overt and well-documented manifestations of structural stigma (Callard et al., 2012) against people with mental illness are segregated housing, some resembling psychiatric institutions (Byrne, 2000; Melnychuk et al., 2009; Metraux et al., 2007; Riley, 2011), and community-wide rejection of mental health facilities (Not-in-My-Backyard) (Piat, 2000). Some supported housing programs also have strict rules that people with mental illness must observe to maintain housing assistance, including prohibition of family or visitors, and mandatory compliance with program requirements or medication regimens (Riley, 2011; Schneider, 2010).

People with mental illness are more likely than others to be counseled to accept a job for which they are overqualified (Wahl, 1999), and they often face increased scrutiny by social workers, educators, physicians, family court administrators, and child protective services personnel (Dolman et al., 2013; Jeffery et al., 2013). On a positive note, NAMI's 2014 review of state legislation found examples of states addressing housing discrimination by enacting rules prohibiting homeless and emergency shelters from refusing services to persons with mental illness and providing funds for home ownership to families of children with disabilities. The NAMI report also documented efforts in some states to increase funding for or make other improvements to supported employment programs (National Alliance on Mental Illness, 2014).

In the arena of higher education, the Americans with Disabilities Act (ADA) and other federal disability laws prohibit discrimination against students with psychiatric disabilities and require that colleges and universities provide them with reasonable accommodations, for example, lighter course loads and extended deadlines. Unfortunately, in U.S. universities, fewer than one in four students with a mental illness will seek treatment or other supportive services (Downs and Eisenberg, 2012). A study of factors that inhibited disclosure of mental illness found these included a high level of self-stigma, fear of future discrimination, having few positive relationships, and sexual minority and Caucasian identity. Previous contact with mental health service users and belief in the effectiveness of treatment were associated with greater likelihood of disclosure and help-seeking (Downs and Eisenberg, 2012).

Another recent survey of campus experiences showed that college students with mental illness reported less social engagement and fewer relationships on campus than the general population, and felt that they were treated differently most of the time. These factors were, in turn, associated with lower graduation rates than the general student population (Salzer, 2012). Research that targets younger populations indicates that earlier experiences have already winnowed down this population, documenting reduced high school graduation rates and lower application rates to higher education (McLeod and Kaiser, 2004). Even when students with mental and/or substance use disorders do seek treatment, they often receive inadequate services, experience delays in obtaining supportive services, face segregation from other students, and receive harsher academic discipline than other students (Livingston, 2013; Losen and Welner, 2001; Skiba and Peterson, 2000; Wald and Losen, 2003).

Although much of the research discussed above referred to people with mental illness, people with substance use disorders also experience structural discrimination in many forms. A national survey of people in recovery from alcohol and drug problems and their families (Hart Research Associates, 2001) documented barriers to treatment, such as lack of insurance and trouble obtaining insurance, the cost of treatment, and lack of access to treatment programs. They also reported fear of discrimination at work and previous experiences of being denied a job or promotion. Despite the hurdles people with substance use disorders face, the implementation of legislation such as the ADA and awarding of federal disability benefits can be more restrictive for people with substance use disorders than for those with mental illness (Join Together, 2003).

Health Care and Treatment Systems

Stigma in the U.S. health care system contributes to disparities in funding for research and treatment of mental disorders in comparison with physical disorders and to the negative attitudes, beliefs, and behaviors of health care professionals toward people with mental and substance use disorders. Structural stigma is manifested in the health care system in the low quality of care for people with mental and substance use disorders and the limited access to behavioral health treatment and other services (Institute of Medicine, 2006; Schulze, 2007; Schulze and Angermeyer, 2003); a fragmented bureaucracy for accessing behavioral health treatment; overuse of coercive approaches to care; and inadequate funding compared with that for physical care (Heflinger and Hinshaw, 2010; Institute of Medicine, 2006; Schomerus and Angermeyer, 2008; Schulze, 2007; Schulze and Angermeyer, 2003).

Parity laws for mental and substance use disorders in the United States have become a cornerstone for efforts to combat the structural inequity of behavioral health coverage versus physical health coverage and to eliminate or reduce coverage restrictions so that behavioral health benefits equate with benefits related to physical health services (Hernandez and Uggen, 2012; Sipe et al., 2015). States with behavioral health parity laws have higher utilization of services among people working for small employers and those in low-income groups (Busch and Barry, 2008). Unfortunately, increased access to care does not necessarily mean increased access to high-quality care or evidence-based treatment.

Recent efforts to address structural stigma in the health care system through parity laws have been accompanied by evolving public attitudes regarding behavioral health in the United States. A 2015 Harris Poll found that close to 90 percent of U.S. adults surveyed considered their mental health and physical health to be equally important, but 56 percent reported that physical health is treated more importantly than mental health in the current health care system, and almost 33 percent thought there were barriers to mental health care in terms of accessibility and cost. In a 2013 survey, 76 percent of adults thought that all health care plans in the United States should be required to include coverage for mental health care (Moniz et al., 2014).

Structural stigma may also be reflected in the de-prioritization and lower levels of funding for behavioral health services and research compared to general physical health services and research, despite the high prevalence of these disorders in the United States and evidence of comparable return on investment (Kelly, 2006; Mark et al., 2014). Research on mental and substance use disorders receives less scientific funding than on physical health conditions (Aoun et al., 2004; Brousseau and Hyman, 2009; Fineberg et al., 2013; Livingston, 2013; Pincus and Fine, 1992). Inadequate investment in behavioral health services research also reduces the availability of evidence-based services, especially in facilities that provide care to the safety net population (Cummings et al., 2013). Quality measurements of behavioral health care amount to only a fraction of physical health care measures, and many are narrowly focused, poorly defined, or lacking in evidence, validation, and meaningfulness (Kilbourne et al., 2010).

Low reimbursements are a factor contributing to the small percentage of psychiatrists who accept insurance (Bishop et al., 2014) and to the persistence of areas with shortages of mental health providers (Cummings et al., 2013). Even with the availability of providers and insurance coverage, insurance benefits have traditionally been more prohibitive of behavioral health services than physical health services, for example, by imposing constraints such as higher deductibles or requiring patients' mental health status to deteriorate before treatment coverage is allowed (Angermeyer et al., 2003; Corrigan et al., 2004a; Livingston, 2013; Muhlbauer, 2002).

Criminal Justice Systems

Structural stigma is apparent in several areas related to the criminal justice system. The disproportionate representation of people with mental illness with criminal justice involvement (Angermeyer et al., 2003; Corrigan et al., 2004b; James and Glaze, 2006; Livingston, 2013; Muhlbauer, 2002; Sarteschi, 2013) and their treatment within the criminal justice system may be indicators of how criminal laws are designed and enforced in such a way as to differentially target and adversely affect people with mental illness. Nationally, more than one-half of jail and prison inmates in 2005 had mental health problems (Angermeyer et al, 2003; Corrigan et al., 2004b; James and Glaze, 2006; Livingston, 2013; Muhlbauer, 2002; Sarteschi, 2013; Teplin et al., 2005). Incarcerated individuals with mental illness were more likely to have experienced multiple arrests and incarcerations, and only one in three people with mental health problems in prisons and less than one in five of those in jails accessed treatment since their imprisonment. Most U.S. states have more people with mental illness in prisons or jails than in state-operated psychiatric hospitals (Torrey et al., 2014).

To counter these trends, 11 states passed legislation in 2014 to halt the inappropriate flow of people with mental illness into the criminal justice system. Strategies included, for example, increasing training programs for law enforcement officers, examining arrests of people with mental illness and developing diversion programs, addressing court systems responses to people with mental illness, and establishing county-level mental health courts (National Alliance on Mental Illness, 2014). In 2004, Congress authorized the Justice and Mental Health Collaboration Program through the Mentally Ill Offender Treatment and Crime Reduction Act. It is a grant program to help states, local governments, and tribal organizations improve responses to people with mental illness in the criminal justice system through collaboration of efforts among the criminal justice, juvenile justice, and mental health and substance use treatment systems. Reauthorized for an additional 5 years in 2008, the act was expanded to address law enforcement responses (Council of State Governments Justice Center, 2015).

In corrections systems, whether prisons or jails, people with mental illness are more frequently abused by staff and inmates (Human Rights Watch, 2015; Wolff et al., 2007); more likely to receive sanctions like solitary confinement (Cloud et al., 2015; James and Glaze, 2006; Subramanian et al., 2015); given longer sentences; and more often denied parole (Livingston, 2013) than inmates without mental illness. While under community supervision, people with mental illness experience more intense supervision and face a higher likelihood of receiving technical violations than others under supervision even though the rate of new offenses is similar between people with and without mental illness (Eno Louden and Skeem, 2013).

The complex relationship between substance use and criminal behavior is beyond the scope of this report. However, in terms of structural stigma, it is important to note that institutional policies that treat substance use disorders primarily as a criminal issue (e.g., the U.S. war on drugs) rather than a health concern have promoted a stigmatizing environment that excludes and marginalizes people with substance use disorders (Bluthenthal et al., 2000; Inciardi, 1986; Livingston, 2012). Antidrug messages and harsh criminal sentences for drug use appear to label people with these disorders as unwanted by society (Rivera et al., 2014). Thus the social processes designed to control substance misuse may actually promote its continuation by increasing shame (Livingston, 2012) and deepen the public and structural stigmatization of this population.

Public Stigma

Public stigma refers to the attitudes of the general public and also to attitudes of subgroups, such as first responders or clergy that may have norms that differ from the general public or other social groups. Public stigma persists in part because structural stigma in the form of laws, regulations and policies appears to endorse prejudice and discrimination against people with behavioral health disorders. A recent systematic review (Parsespe and Cabbassa, 2013) identified 36 articles published over the last 25 years that reported on results from population-based studies of public stigma in the United States. Many of the articles were secondary analyses of findings from national surveys, including the National Comorbidity Survey-Replication and the GSS's National Stigma Studies. These surveys examined public stigma toward people with a broad array of disorders, including adults with depression, schizophrenia, alcohol or drug dependency and children with depression, attention-deficit hyperactivity disorder, and oppositional defiant disorder.

The results of this review, confirmed by other researchers, indicate that public stigma leads to social segregation as well as diminished self-efficacy in people with mental and substance use disorders (Corrigan and Shapiro, 2010; Parcesepe and Cabassa, 2013; Pescosolido et al., 2007). Stigmatizing beliefs about the competency of people with mental illness compromise these individuals' financial autonomy, restrict opportunities, and may lead to coercive treatment, such as mandatory participation in treatment (Corrigan and Shapiro, 2010; Pescosolido et al., 2007). Despite the importance of social support for the recovery of those with substance use disorders, stigma instead contributes to social exclusion (Room, 2005). Also of importance, stigma may affect not only the substance user but his or her family members and friends as well (Corrigan et al., 2006a). Over time in both the United States and other countries, knowledge about mental and substance use disorders is increasing, but issues related to social exclusion also remain high (Pescosolido et al., 2007, 2010).

Self-Stigma

As people with mental and substance use disorders become aware of public stigma and of related discriminatory practices, they internalize the perceived stigma and apply it to themselves. The effects of self-stigma include lowered self-esteem, decreased self-efficacy, and psychologically harmful feelings of embarrassment and shame. Low self-esteem and low self-efficacy can lead to what Corrigan refers to as the "why try" effect, meaning why should a person try to live and work independently if he or she is not valued (Corrigan et al., 2009a).

Among people with mental and substance use disorders, low self-efficacy is associated with failure to pursue work or independent living; a greater degree of self-esteem is associated with goal attainment (e.g., symptom reduction, financial and academic problems), quality of life (e.g., satisfaction with work, housing, health, and finance), and help-seeking behavior (Corrigan et al., 2009b). A substantial body of research has shown that there is a negative relationship between stigma and help-seeking (Clement et al., 2015; Corrigan et al., 2014). Self-stigma can also be a barrier to recovery and community integration.

People who have disclosed their experiences report lower levels of self-stigma (Chinman et al., 2014). In a systematic review of research published between 1980 and 2011 examining associations between mental health-related stigma and help-seeking for mental health problems, Clement and colleagues (2015) found that stigma related to fears about the consequences of disclosure was the fourth highest ranked barrier to help-seeking. Members of racial and ethnic minorities, youth, men, military service members, and health professionals were disproportionately deterred from seeking help by fears of being stigmatized. In addition, the level of public stigma shaped both reported experiences of stigma, self-stigma, and an unwillingness to use services (Evans-Lacko et al., 2012a; Mojtabai, 2010).

Stigma against children and adolescents is a serious concern because of its negative impacts, including decreased feelings of self-worth and willingness to enter treatment, and because of the deleterious long-term effects of untreated mental or substance use disorders. Compared with the adult population, stigma against children with mental disorders is less well studied. A 2010 review of studies of stigma related to childhood mental disorders concluded that stigma research lacked conceptual underpinnings and that the evidence base was quite sparse (Mukolo et al., 2010).

The National Stigma Study-Children, which was the first to include a nationally representative sample of participants to examine public stigma of childhood mental disorders specifically focused on attention-deficit/hyperactivity disorder (ADHD) and depression, comparing public attitudes and knowledge of these disorders with asthma or "daily troubles." One set of analyses showed that 81 percent of the adult sample perceived children with depression to be dangerous to themselves or others, compared with children who had asthma or "daily troubles" (Pescosolido et al., 2007). A smaller but substantial proportion (33%) also perceived children with ADHD to be dangerous. Large proportions of the sample thought that children and adolescents with mental health problems would likely experience rejection at school (45%) and would experience stigma into adulthood (43%). Many respondents also had negative views of the benefits of medication (Pescosolido et al., 2007). The researchers concluded that some public beliefs about mental illness and treatment were based on a lack of accurate information and could present barriers for providers and for parents and others who seek treatment (Pescosolido et al., 2008a).

A growing body of research focuses on young people's subjective experiences of stigma. Interviews with 56 adolescents in a midwestern U.S. city found that 62 percent of youth experienced stigma with peers; 46 percent reported feeling stigmatized by their families; and 35 percent reported experiencing fear, dislike, avoidance, and underestimation of their abilities by school staff (Moses, 2010).

In a study of 40 adolescents taking psychiatric medication for a diagnosed mental illness, 90 percent reported experience of at least one stigma construct of secrecy, shame, and limited social interaction (Kranke et al., 2010). The study also found that adolescents' perceptions of the norms of family members and school environments can increase their experience of stigma or protect against it. Results of a large study of youth in Australia suggested that using accurate psychiatric labels reduces stigma and may assist youth by reducing perceptions of weakness (Wright et al., 2011).

The Web-based Injury Statistics Query and Reporting System (WISQARS™) shows that suicide is the second leading cause of death among young people in the United States aged 15 to 34 years (Centers for Disease Control and Prevention, 2015). There is strong evidence that stigma is an impediment to help-seeking on the part of young people and their families. Studies of family engagement in treatment have provided insight into how stigma poses barriers to care. A review of 12 qualitative studies in the United Kingdom on factors that facilitate or inhibit access and engagement in parenting programs for children with disruptive behavior problems pointed to factors directly or indirectly related to stigma (Koerting et al., 2013). Stigma was one of the factors that emerged as a prominent barrier to service from the perspective of both parents and professionals. In these studies, stigma was manifested as shame about needing help, perceived parental failure, and fear of being labeled. Lack of information and lack of awareness about services were also major barriers to accessing care. Mainly from the professionals' perspectives, one of the main facilitators of access was effective advertisement and service promotion using media, such as leaflets or posters in locations visited by parents, promotion on the internet, local newspapers, radio stations, newsletters, and parenting forums.

TARGETS AND INTERVENTIONS TO ADDRESS STIGMA

In subsequent chapters of the report, the committee reviews the evidence on the effectiveness of stigma reduction interventions and approaches. In this section, we provide an overview of the potential targets and interventions that emerged from the committee's examination of the factors influencing each type of stigma and its consequences. Figure 2-1 illustrates the relationships among consequences of stigma at various levels and potential targets and interventions to reduce stigma at each level.

As shown in Figure 2-1, targets of structural stigma would include legislators, institutions, and policy makers of systems and organizations that fund and regulate the places and situations where discrimination, lack of opportunities, and lack of access to quality treatment persist. The interventions that would be appropriate for this level are legal, policy, advocacy, and professional education strategies. Strategies would be aimed at changing decision-making processes, policies, and regulations that support discrimination against people with mental and substance use disorders.

Targets for interventions to reduce public stigma include the general public and landlords, employers, health care providers, and groups within the criminal justice system. The corresponding interventions would be aimed at changing behaviors and interactions from discrimination, fear, neglect, and sometimes abuse to extending support, high-quality treatment, and equal opportunities for housing, employment, and personal success. Examples of such interventions include use of media for mass messaging to dispel myths regarding behavioral health disorders and treatment, education to counter the lack of knowledge about disorders and treatment, contact with people with behavioral disorders, and protest strategies against discrimination.

The general effects of self-stigma and the "why try" effect may be diminished by interventions that target individuals with behavioral disorders. As shown in Figure 2-1, such interventions would focus on promoting self-esteem and self-efficacy; empowerment through peer support, mentoring, and education to dispel myths and increase social and coping skills; and education to encourage treatment engagement (Corrigan et al., 2009a). Treatment engagement is significant because evidence-based treatments have been shown to facilitate recovery by promoting behaviors, such as symptom monitoring, continuing to take prescribed medications, and seeking out supported employment opportunities; and by encouraging family interventions, increasing skills related to illness management, and promoting entry into integrated treatment for mental and substance use disorders (Corrigan et al., 2009a, 2009b, 2014). For many individuals, disclosure may be an initial step in the process of reducing self-stigma when it can be done in a safe and strategic manner (Bos et al., 2009; Corrigan and Rao, 2012).

Chapter 4 will review the growing evidence base on the effectiveness of these types of intervention strategies as approaches to reducing stigma at each of the major levels.

3

The Science of Communication

This chapter describes a communications framework that attends to the behavioral and cognitive principles that would drive the selection of targets, messages, and delivery methods of an effective anti-stigma initiative. The chapter provides details about reaching specific target audiences for future campaigns that have been selected through a prioritizing process that includes stakeholder participation and is informed by relevant theory and formative research.

BACKGROUND

To change health-related public norms and behaviors, public health organizations often partner with communication scientists. The most effective and long lasting of these collaborative efforts have been based on communications science and informed by behavioral theory (Institute of Medicine, 2002). Health-related behavior is influenced by a range of structural, social, and psychological factors, which include access to health-related resources, prevalent social norms, and personal agency and intentions. Communication strategies can influence all of these factors, and communications strategies and communication science perspectives are relevant across structural, public, and self-stigma.

Historically, efforts to promote public perception of mental and substance use disorders as treatable diseases have been successful, but these efforts have not led to a general reduction of public stigma related to these disorders. Efforts to promote the perception of mental and substance use disorders as diseases like any others have taken a mental health literacy approach. Mental health literacy campaigns are educational efforts aimed at improving understanding of behavioral health disorders, and their prevention and treatment (Jorm, 2012). Efforts to improve the public's understanding of mental illness as a disease have been successful in reducing attributional stigma, that is, the belief that people are to blame for their behavioral health problems (Corrigan, 2004; Pescosolido et al., 2013), but blaming persists in regard to substance use disorders. The biogenic view of the origins of mental illness and addiction can discourage punitive attitudes and coercive approaches to treatment, and encourage sympathetic attitudes, and support of recovery-oriented treatment and rehabilitative services (Corrigan, 2004). However, this approach has also produced unintended consequences by bringing attention to the "differentness" of people with and without these disorders (Kvaale et al., 2013a, 2013b). This is a concern since one of the ultimate goals of anti-stigma campaigns is to promote attitudes of inclusion regarding people with mental and substance use disorders.

An added concern is that, while public health communications campaigns may increase public knowledge about mental and substance use disorders, changing behavior toward people with these disorders typically requires additional change in what is believed, felt, and desired in terms of outcomes. Habitual and unconscious behaviors are particularly difficult to change as are behaviors that are motivated by unquestioned social norms and/or strong emotions such as fear (Institute of Medicine, 2002). This may partly explain the persistence of the stereotype of dangerousness and unpredictability.

Communication efforts built on a foundation of behavioral theory will identify which public norms and behaviors to target, structure the message to be remembered so as to have lasting impact, and facilitate selection of the best message platform or source. The goal of stigma change efforts may be to reduce stigmatizing beliefs and behaviors or reinforce positive attitudes. Science-based communication campaigns to change stigma must begin by identifying the range of attitudes and beliefs in the general public, or within smaller target audiences, and determine which of those attitudes, beliefs, and/or behaviors should be targeted for change and which might be positive in influence and thus targeted for reinforcement.

Other essential steps in the planning include choice of target audience(s), behavioral objectives, a message strategy and implementation, and evaluation of plans. Activities in the planning phase include choosing which channels and settings will be used for message dissemination, conducting formative research and ongoing monitoring, and evaluation to support the effort (Institute of Medicine, 2002). Following these steps helps to increase the effectiveness of behavioral health communication efforts in meeting campaign goals and objectives (Institute of Medicine, 2002). The next section will detail these steps and focus on how communication science principles and perspectives can be applied within a campaign to change behavioral health social norms and behaviors.

SETTING GOALS FOR BEHAVIOR CHANGE

Before attempting to identify a target audience, intervention designers must have a thoughtful discussion informed by stakeholder input about what specific behaviors they want to change or reinforce, based on scientific evidence linking those behaviors to a stated outcome related to the goals and objectives of the campaign (Institute of Medicine, 2002). An important consideration is the feasibility of the behavior or behavioral change—is it one that the potential target populations can reasonably perform? For example, asking someone to break laws to change their behavior is not tenable. The desired behavior change must also be specific, for example, a vague categorical directive to "eat healthier" rarely produces results, whereas a specific behavior change goal, such as "walk for at least 30 minutes a day" or "eat two additional servings of fruits or vegetables a day," is more likely to result in behavior change (Institute of Medicine, 2002). Finally, it's important to be realistic and specific about the timeframe over which the behavior change will be assessed and how the related success in meeting campaign objectives will be evaluated. Behavior change rarely happens quickly so a message that is delivered multiple times on a consistent and ongoing basis is more likely to change behavior in a lasting way than a one-time action (Institute of Medicine, 2002).

REACHING TARGET AUDIENCES

The source, the message, the platform, and the production features of the intervention will vary with the target audience and the goals of the intervention. A well-tailored message that is designed for a specific audience increases the likelihood of success in meeting project goals and objectives. This section will identify potential target audiences for stigma change and focus on the goals of the messages for various target audiences. There are many potential target audiences campaign designers might choose to focus on in a given campaign, and the examples provided here should not be considered comprehensive or exclusive. These examples are provided to guide campaign designers through the audience selection and message design processes and should not be used in place of formative research.

Among the stakeholders involved in stigma change efforts, there are many independent and sometimes mutually conflicting agendas. Likewise, an appreciation for the diversity of the U.S. public and the basic principles of communication science make clear that there cannot be a single target audience in our national efforts to reduce behavioral health stigma. Because stigma comes from many sources, there will be many targets on the receiving end of anti-stigma messages. Primary targets for stigma change campaigns include policy makers who have the ability to change laws that enable structural stigma against people with mental and substance use disorders; employers and landlords who have the power to deny livelihoods and housing to people with these disorders; mental health workers whose job is to provide nonjudgmental, culturally competent, evidence-based treatment; people with mental and substance use disorders who self-stigmatize in ways that reduce their quality of life; and the general public who can discriminate against or support and empower people with behavioral health disorders, notably through their support or opposition to policy, regulation, and legislation concerning people with mental and substance use disorders.

In addition to being diverse, potential target audiences are sometimes difficult to define. Targeting the full range of audiences with sufficient frequency would require a significant commitment of time and resources. Audience segmentation is a classic approach to choosing how best to focus and stage communication efforts and a necessary step in the process of design and development of communication campaigns (Atkin and Freimuth, 1989; Grunig, 1989; Rogers and Storey, 1987; Slater et al., 1997). Segmentation is a process by which a heterogeneous population is partitioned into subgroups or segments of people with similar needs, experiences, and/or other characteristics (Institute of Medicine, 2002); for example, we might segment high school students from college students when crafting messages about suicide. Audiences whose personal values and priorities resonate with a message process the message more deeply, remember it better, and are more likely to act on the message than an audience to whom the message is not so relevant (Institute of Medicine, 2002). Audience segmentation is most effective when it accurately identifies subaudiences for whom a particular message is relevant and distinguishes them from those for whom it is not relevant. Ultimately, the goal is to maximize the relevance of a message by targeting it to the audience most receptive to it.

An important precursor to detailed formative research for each target population is the discussion of the specific types of desired outcomes, such as awareness, belief change, or behavioral change. In the case of stigma change, this includes a need to understand how the potential audience contributes to stigma; for example, do they have a role in supporting a loved one who experiences stigma first hand, or are they able to influence structural stigma from a leadership or decision-making position? Communication campaigns tend to fail for two reasons—failure to identify well-defined goals and objectives for the campaign (Kirby et al., 2001) and failure to reach the intended audience(s) in a sustained or adequately frequent manner (Snyder et al., 2004). Potential target audiences and related goals and objectives for stigma change campaigns are discussed briefly below.

Federal Legislators and State Law Makers

Legislators have considerable influence over the distribution of funding for mental health and substance use services and other social policies that influence the lives of people with mental and substance use disorders. Policy and decision makers who have negative attitudes toward people with mental illness may choose to block funding for services while those who hold positive attitudes may direct resources toward supportive services. In the case of policy makers, the ultimate goal may be a change in public norms and behaviors by reducing stigma at the structural level through the sponsorship and enactment of antidiscrimination or other supportive policies and laws. Objectives related to this goal would focus on preliminary steps aimed at changing the target audience's beliefs about people with mental and substance use disorders or the nature of the disorders. Desired outcomes would be that legislators and decision makers develop more awareness of relevant issues, including better understanding of behavioral health disorders and related stigma, and greater empathy for people with these disorders. Decision makers must also come to believe and agree as a group that change is possible and needed. To enact change, legislators and decision makers must first form the intent to act, which requires creation of a positive attitude toward the act of creating a new policy. Once policy goals for reducing structural stigma have been established, formative research needs to identify key policy makers and characteristics that they have in common to set the stage for targeted and effective messaging.

Employers and Landlords

As noted earlier in this report, people with mental illness and substance use disorders are often perceived as being dangerous and unpredictable (Link et al., 1992, 1999a, 1999b). The high rates of unemployment, homelessness, and housing discrimination observed among people with mental illness and addiction are among the consequences of this stereotype. Consequently, employers and landlords are important target audiences for anti-stigma messaging. In this case, the ultimate goal is to increase the hiring of peple with mental illness and to increase willingness to rent to people with mental illness. Employers and landlords are a relatively amorphous target audience. Formative research would need to be done in specific neighborhoods and communities to identify the targets for the messages. General characteristics might be established on the basis of research in one or two markets to allow for the development of messages, choice of platform(s) for delivery, and completion of other steps in the communications process outlined above. The messages could then be adapted and scaled-up for delivery in multiple employment and housing markets.

Younger Audiences

The increasing popularity of nontraditional media among young people has led to considerations of new ways to reach them. Although past efforts to combat stigma against mental and substance use disorders have typically relied on traditional print, and television-based media campaigns, in recent years both researchers and anti-stigma campaign designers have turned toward the internet and social media to deploy anti-stigma efforts, collect previously unavailable data, and track the influence of these contemporary media platforms on stigma. A recent review by Moorhead and colleagues (2013) systematically examined 98 studies on the influence of social media for health communication. They identified six key benefits to using social media in health communications: increased interaction with others; more available, shared, and tailored information; increased accessibility and widening access to health information; peer and social support; public health surveillance; and potential to influence health policy (Moorhead et al., 2013).

Young adults often turn to the internet to find support from like-minded peers on family and relationship problems and mental health concerns, such as depression, drug and alcohol use, eating disorders, and suicidality (Fukkink, 2011). Increasingly, formalized peer support programs are being established online. One example is the Dutch Share in Trust Project, which trains young adults (ages 16-23) to serve as peer counselors in a supportive online chat (Fukkink, 2011). Although research on this type of online support is still in its early stages, preliminary evidence suggests that young people may successfully provide positive socioemotional support for one another online (Fukkink, 2011).

In an effort to counter misinformation that is online and bring accurate, nonstigmatizing messages to the forefront, behavioral health organizations can use advertisements and search- engine optimization strategies to bring accurate and professional health resources to the top of internet search results (Birnbaum et al., 2014). In addition, when designing educational online resources, campaign planners need to partner with young adults to help ensure that messages are engaging, appealing, and developmentally appropriate to the adolescents who are likely to seek information (Birnbaum et al., 2014).

In addition to online mental health forums, Twitter is increasingly used to replace stereotypes with the "real face" of mental illness. During one online protest of an offensive "mental patient" Halloween costume, Twitter users posted "lived experience selfies" with accompanying text that said, "This is what a real mental patient looks like" (Betton et al., 2015, pp. 443-444). As technology evolves, so do the potential platforms by which people with mental and substance use disorders can share their experiences.

Health Care Professionals

Health care workers' attitudes and beliefs regarding the nature of mental and substance use disorders influence the treatment they provide to people with these disorders for both behavioral and somatic conditions (Keane, 1991; Levey and Howells, 1994). For example, in a review of articles about attitudes among emergency department caregivers, Clark and colleagues (2014) found that staff in those departments commonly reported feeling challenged by mental health problems, angry and fearful about aggressive or unusual behavior, and frustrated by what they saw as a "revolving door" of repeat admissions. However, staff who had been educated and trained in treating mental disorders were better able to engage with the patients and more likely to convey messages about hope and recovery.

Interventions directed at medical students have found that attitudes are more amenable to change early in their education and training, and that these attitudes tend to solidify as students progress through medical school and residency (Papish et al., 2013). Formative research can help to identify the specific attitudes and beliefs that prompt a subgroup of health care providers to stigmatize their clientele. So, for example, since research indicates that the stereotype of dangerousness and unpredictability is prevalent among health professionals (Levey and Howells, 1994), the objectives of an anti-stigma intervention for this audience would focus on improving mental health literacy about the relationships between violence and behavioral disorders, and increasing empathetic responses and decreasing aversive responses to people with mental or substance use disorders.

People with Mental and Substance Use Disorders

Self-stigma negatively influences decisions about seeking treatment and following regimens of care. Research in this area suggests that self-stigma is decreased after "coming out" as a person with mental illness and/or disclosing related experiences (Corrigan et al., 2013). Disclosure may elicit both affective change (more self-pride, self-worth, and hope) and cognitive change (knowledge that effective treatment exists and recovery is possible). To reach this audience and encourage selective disclosure or facilitate contact with someone who is already "out," campaign designers should conduct formative, community-level research to identify local community resources. Community clinics and schools could be valuable hubs of information to get the word out via print materials such as posters and advertisements containing well-crafted messages. Additionally, high-profile individuals with mental illness and/or substance use disorders may be particularly effective in reducing self-stigma and encouraging selective disclosure.

Media Professionals

The role of media in perpetuating mental illness and addictions stigma is an important target for stigma change efforts (McGinty et al., 2014). The goals of communication targeted toward media professionals would be to educate them about appropriate language to use to describe mental illness and substance use disorders, to increase their sensitivity when covering behavioral health issues in the news, and to produce more balanced and fact-based reporting of violent events that involve people with serious behavioral health problems. The messages would have to get their attention, be remembered, and model appropriate behavior change, that is, the desired modifications in their reporting.

CHOOSING A MESSAGE SOURCE

The source that delivers the behavioral health messages has a strong impact on how messages are received, for example, whether messages are perceived as credible, meaningful, and relevant. The choice of a source needs to be made after the audience is selected because the source needs to be someone whom the target audience finds relevant and worthy of trust and respect. This may be someone the audience relates to or knows personally, someone who represents the target audience, a recognizable celebrity or public figure, someone whom the target audience regards as an influential role model, or someone who is friendly and anonymous, such as a fictional or animated character (Weinreich, 1999).

Every communication has a source either stated by the designer or inferred by the audience. Sources can be both proximal and/or distal. The distal source is the organization sponsoring the message. The proximal source is the person delivering the message. The proximal source generally has more powerful effects than the distal source, although trusted and distrusted distal sources can create a halo of credibility or lack thereof. The influence of proximal sources is greater in visual, audio, and audiovisual media, but there are exceptions to this rule. Text and print messages have both distal and proximal sources, and, in some cases, the distal source is more influential than the proximal source. For example, a well-known distal source such as a newspaper (e.g., the *New York Times*) may be more influential than the proximal source, the journalist(s) named in the byline.

A robust body of research suggests that people who are living successfully and openly with mental or substance use disorders are extremely powerful proximal sources (Borschmann et al., 2014; Corrigan et al., 2012; Griffiths et al., 2014; James and Glaze, 2006; Yamaguchi et al., 2013). From a communication science point of view, this is because they embody the message "I have a mental illness and I am like you. I have a life and a job, and I experience both good things and bad things." As proximal sources, peers offer positive images and proof of concept all in one package. Audiences are likely to attribute them with high credibility because they have insider knowledge and experience.

People are more receptive to sources that are similar to themselves, and to people who embody characteristics, such as likeability, expertise, and trustworthiness. Message sources for target audiences should be selected with these characteristics in mind, and evaluative research can help identify the best choices among alternatives. For example, for legislators and policy makers, those in similar jobs (lawyers, administrators) with lived experience might be excellent choices. For the general public, an effective campaign might include many different sources from various demographic groups sending the same message. For example, landlords could be a message source for fellow landlords, and journalists, especially those with lived experience of mental or substance use disorders, could be the source of messages sent to other journalists.

MESSAGE GOALS AND DESIGNS

Once a target audience, a source, and objectives have been established, communication planning turns to the design of the message. The message should be specific, focused, and limited in scope. A message typically contains one main idea that is related to the campaign objectives (Ferguson, 1999). An effective message achieves the producer's goals, which typically include capturing attention, holding the audience's memory for information, gaining acceptance, and ultimately changing attitudes, changing behavioral intentions, or changing behavior.

Several principles guide message design at both the macro and micro levels. Effective messages are argumentatively strong and engage the audience's mental and emotional resources. Argumentatively strong messages are ones that generate mostly favorable thoughts (as opposed to unfavorable thoughts) in the target audience. Formative and evaluative research is necessary to craft argumentatively strong appeals to the target audience, but most argumentatively strong messages are ones that argue from the consequences to the targets of change (O'Keefe, 2013).

Formative and evaluative research is needed to guide the construction and testing of such arguments for the target audience, but what makes a message strong is that it highlights personal consequences that are salient to the targeted audience. This idea is simple and sounds common sensical but campaigns often fail by ignoring it. Such failure is usually due to one or more of the following reasons: (1) the message design was not driven by testing, (2) the message focused on consequences but not relevant personal ones, (3) the message focused on personal consequences but failed to test which were most salient in the target audience, and (4) the argument that was crafted did not fit with the desired campaign outcome. A carefully designed communication campaign would use a clear and well-defined methodology with specific goals and direct application to the communication campaigns. The Food and Drug Administration used such a methodology to design the first generation of its The Real Cost campaign.[1] When exposed to a message through one or more media outlets, focusing attention to the message's content will require engaging the audience both emotionally and cognitively. A variety of message features can gain and sustain an audience's attention. Two features are particularly effective: the use of stories (i.e., narrative forms of information) and testimony (i.e., testimonial cases as exemplars) (Kim et al., 2012; Kreuter et al., 2007; Zillmann and Brosius, 2012). To ensure that core ideas and information remain mentally available to the target audience, communications strategies need to include well-crafted narratives and/or exemplars that deliver strong arguments and provide information in a form that is engaging, comprehensible, and memorable or mentally "sticky."

For example, if the goal is to understand the specifics about why landlords do not want to rent to people with mental illness, intervention planners might conduct formative research that shows it is because the landlords think tenants with mental illness will not pay their rent and will damage the apartment. A message might provide information about the

---

[1]For more information about The Real Cost campaign, see http://therealcost.betobaccofree.hhs.gov/costs/index.html [March 2016].

proportion of renters with mental illness who pay rent on time or exemplars of such people successfully living in a variety of types of rental properties. Although numbers matter, research suggests that exemplars are stickier and more likely to determine what is remembered and believed.

Similarly, if the target audience is policy or decision makers and the goal is to change a law forbidding a certain action by a person with a mental illness, for example, holding public office, the message designers would want to know first if the law exists as a forgotten remnant on the books and most decision makers are unaware of it or if there is a current belief among the policy and decisions makers that people with mental illnesses are not capable of holding a public office. In the first case, raising the policy and decision makers' awareness of the discriminatory law may be all that is necessary. In the second case, a message would be designed to convince the target audience that what they currently know and/or believe about people with mental illnesses is not accurate. At the same time, the goal would be to change the policy and decision makers' affective stance from one of fear and doubt to one of calm and positive belief in the capabilities of people with mental illnesses.

As another example, efforts to encourage more balanced media coverage of mental illness and substance use disorders, along with related and tragic events including suicide and gun violence, could include programs that provide constructive feedback to journalists about how to cover issues related to mental health. Giving journalists alternatives and resources to inform their reporting is crucial. FactCheck.org,[2] an online program sponsored by the Annenberg Public Policy Center is example of a program of this type. It provides journalists with data and information on the deleterious consequences of negative coverage and false political ads along with techniques about how to cover false and negative ads.

MAKING THE MOST OF THE MESSAGE

Message structure and content influence attention, cognition, emotion, and intentions. In designing a message, the producer can capture the audience's attention, improve the audience's recollection of the message, and elicit emotional responses through the use of structural features that work in accordance with people's cognitive and physiological processes.

When designing audio and video messages, producers can direct audience attention to focus on specific moments and specific contents by designing messages with structural features that elicit orienting responses. An orienting response is a set of physiological responses (i.e., turning one's sensory receptors toward the new event, decrease in heart

---

[2]For more information about FactCheck.org, see http://www.factcheck.org/ [March 2016].

rate, and increase in skin temperature and conductance) to things that are novel, or signal personally relevant information to the viewer (Graham, 1979). Examples of structural features in a message that elicit an orienting response include a change from sound to silence, scene changes, camera changes, movement from off screen to on screen, movement toward a still camera, changes from one voice to another, animation, and pop-up windows. The specific advantage of using such structural features is they are known to increase attention to the message for approximately 2 seconds, and in particular to draw attention to the feature that elicited the viewer's orienting response (Lang, 1990; Lang et al., 2002, 2013b).

In addition to manipulating audience attention through structural features, the content of a message can also be used to focus attention in a specific moment. Motivationally relevant content presents an opportunity or a threat, elicits either an appetitive or aversive response, or corresponds with an individual learned motivator that has been developed and held over time. Introducing motivationally relevant content, images, or sounds increases audience attention and holds that attention as long as the motivationally relevant material is on screen (Lang, 2006; Lang et al., 2013a). Message producers should carefully consider which content they include and whether it stimulates an appetitive or aversive response in the audience. For example, when designing a message aimed at people with substance use disorders, producers should avoid including images of the substance (e.g., avoid including a picture of alcohol in a message aimed at alcoholics) as it can elicit both an orienting response and appetitive motivational activation that can result in attention and positive emotion to the substance, which would be an unintended negative response contrary to the objectives of the message and the goals of the campaign.

It is possible to maintain audience attention throughout an entire message. One approach is an expansion of the use of structural features. Incorporating orienting response-eliciting structural features at a rate of five or more per 30 seconds will produce steady attention that is maintained over that period of time. Another approach is to use a narrative (a chronological presentation of information) and ensure that the message tells a story with a clear beginning, middle, and end (Lang, 1989; Lang et al., 2000; Schneider, 2004). When using a narrative, it is also important to include emotionally relevant material throughout the message.

Although it may seem straightforward to control audience attention through the structural features of a message, the limits of human cognitive processing ability force message producers to make decisions about how many and which features to use. Memory is always a tradeoff with increasing structural and content complexity—when content is complex, there is a need to simplify structure, and when structure is complex, there is a need to simplify content. For example, orienting responses increase memory if the thing one wants people to remember is the thing that elicited the orienting response (Lang et al., 2002) and if there is sufficient time to encode the thing one wants remembered. Thus, for a complex message, producers will need to devote more time and use fewer structural features (Lang et al., 1993). A message containing more complex content will require more time to encode it into memory, and a complex message will not be remembered as well when it is paired with fast-changing sounds, scenes, and animations.

Motivationally relevant material increases memory for specific moments or things if the thing that is motivationally relevant is the thing you want remembered, and if the motivationally relevant thing is integrated with the information you want remembered rather than simply co-occurring (Sparks and Lang, 2014). In the context of the example above, images of substances and paraphernalia in a message may lead to the unintended consequence of strengthening memory for positive feelings associated with substance use.

In some cases, a message producer may want the audience to remember having seen the message but not particulars of its content. In this scenario, the producer would use many orienting response-eliciting structural features (more than 10 in 30 seconds) and many different types of orienting and eliciting structural functions in multiple channels (Grabe et al., 2000). To promote recollection of the message but not all the content, the producer can use arousing negative emotional material (Lang et al., 1996, 2007). In these approaches, people will remember the arousing negative material and the information that follows it; however, their memory for the preceding information will be poor.

To increase memory for the message and its contents, producers need to consider the quality of the emotion. Positive emotion widens focus and memory while negative emotion narrows focus and memory (Yegiyan and Yonelinas, 2011). Producers can also use narratives to simplify message processing (Lang, 1989; Schneider, 2004). Using orienting response-eliciting structural features at a rate of about five to seven per 30 seconds and placing them so that important information follows them and is available for at least 3 seconds is a good way to increase memory (Lang et al., 2014a, 2014b). Using audio and video (multiple channel) redundancy, especially for important points, also increases memory (Lang, 1995).

Although messages with negative appeals can compel attention and capture memory, message designers should be cautious when using them. After viewing a message with a negative appeal, people will remember the negative thing very well, and they will have decent memory for things that followed it, but they will not remember things in the message that preceded it (Newhagen and Reeves, 1992). In this case, message designers need to pay particular attention to the priorities of the content before and after the negative appeal to decide accordingly. Moreover, people may engage in defensive processing, which results in low attention, poor memory, and dislike for the message (Witte and Allen, 2000). Message producers can make their message more likable by choosing attractive, familiar sources with friendly and dominant personalities who are polite, flatter the message recipient, and criticize with caution.

Messages that are not perceived as credible will not be effective, but producers can increase the credibility of messages by using sources that are likeable, and if appropriate, expert in the field (Reeves and Nass, 1996). People with the lived experience of behavioral health problems will be particularly credible sources. Credibility is further bolstered by presenting strong arguments in words and weak arguments in pictures (Lang and Yegiyan, 2008) as well as by using camera techniques that look "up" at the source (Reeves and Nass, 1996). Men are unfairly perceived as more credible than women, but message producers can use this to their advantage if they choose to do so (Reeves and Nass, 1996).

Message producers can draw on the automatic activation of human motivational systems to enhance the efficacy of messages. For example, pictures elicit greater motivational activation and larger biological imperatives (i.e., the motivation to approach or avoid the stimulus) than words while words reduce biological imperatives and increase thinking (Lang et al., 2015). If there is something one wants the message recipient to like or to do, a good approach is to associate the desired action with something they already enjoy doing (Lang et al., 2014b). Likewise, to steer people away from a particular attitude or behavior, associate the action in question with something the viewer already dislikes (Lang et al., 2014a). Finally, by using positive and negative emotions sequentially in messages, the producer can increase the viewer's memory for messages (Keene, 2014; Thorson and Friestad, 1989). One final consideration for message producers is that pictures are more likely to shift implicit attitudes and words are more likely to affect thoughtful opinions or the viewer's explicit attitudes. Used together, these techniques can create a message that affects behavior and attitude across multiple levels and domains.

CHOOSING THE MEDIUM BASED ON THE TARGET

Once a message is designed, the producers need to take steps to ensure that it is received as intended by the target audience. On the most basic level, messages that are not perceived are not effective, so the first requirement is that messages need to get to the target. Producers should consider which platforms will best reach their target. When presented with the choice of channels (i.e., social media, telephone calls, etc.), three questions should be asked: (1) What messages can be sent through a particular channel? (2) How is each channel perceived by the audience? and (3) When multiple channels are present, how do they interact in their effects? (Institute of Medicine, 2002).

The list of potential communication channels below are examples and starting points for message producers to consider. This list should not be thought of as comprehensive or fixed.

- *For legislators and policy makers,* face-to-face approaches might be best, followed by a letter or e-mail or a telephone call.
- *For landlords,* good approaches might include mail, e-mail, and social media, which are used by many apartment complexes.
- *For employers,* face-to-face workplace interventions have been shown to be effective (Stuart et al., 2014a, 2014b).
- *For people with behavioral health problems,* face-to-face interaction with people with lived experience is best (Borschmann et al., 2014; Corrigan et al., 2012). Social media sites for people with lived experience are another possibility.
- *For health care workers,* there are many avenues for messaging, including workplace informational materials; continuing education; face-to-face contact with people with lived experiences, especially those who are health professionals; and billboards near health care facilities and on buses and trains along routes that workers might use to get to work.
- *For journalists,* there are also many avenues for messaging including professional conferences; journalism fellowships; curriculum in journalism schools; online guidelines and materials; and face-to-face contact with persons with lived experiences, especially those who are journalists.

4

Approaches to Reducing Stigma

This chapter describes other national and large-scale anti-stigma interventions that have been implemented and evaluated. They include three major ongoing or completed anti-stigma interventions from Australia, Canada, and England that have been evaluated with reference to the targets, goals, and outcomes, as well as the level of stigma they addressed—structural, public, and or self—and the intervention type, that is, whether it involved protest and advocacy, education, and direct contact or contact-based education. When relevant information is available, the descriptions of the interventions also include a discussion of both their intended outcomes and unintended consequences. As noted above, the dearth of data on what works to reduce stigma is particularly acute as it relates to substance use disorders, and it is not always clear that findings related to mental illness can be generalized to substance use disorders, or even applied across all mental disorders.

APPROACHES AND STRATEGIES

Education

Educational anti-stigma interventions present factual information about the stigmatized condition with the goal of correcting misinformation or contradicting negative attitudes and beliefs. They counter inaccurate stereotypes or myths by replacing them with factual information. An example would be an education campaign to counter the idea that people with mental illness are violent murderers by presenting statistics showing that homicide rates are similar among people with mental illness and the general public (Corrigan et al., 2012). Most of the evidence on educational interventions has been on stigma related to mental illness rather than substance use disorders.

Educational campaigns can be designed for any scale, from local to national, which may explain the status of education interventions as the best-evaluated stigma change tactic (Griffiths et al., 2014; Quinn et al., 2014). Although generally aimed at combating public stigma, educational interventions have been found to be effective in reducing self-stigma, improving stress management, and boosting self-esteem when delivered as a component of cognitive and behavioral therapy (Cook et al., 2014; Heijnders and Van Der Meij, 2006). They have also been effective in acceptance and commitment therapy (Corrigan et al., 2013), an intervention that uses acceptance and mindfulness strategies, together with commitment and behavior change strategies, to change values about mental health and illness (see Hayes et al., 2006).

Evidence is mixed on the effectiveness of educational interventions in changing public stigma in a significant and lasting way (Corrigan et al., 2012, 2015a; Griffiths et al., 2014). For example, Scotland's See Me campaign aimed to correct inaccurate portrayals of mental illness in an effort to normalize the public to mental illness. Surveys conducted 2 years after the start of the campaign showed an 11 percent drop in the expressed belief that the public should be better protected from people with mental health problems and a 17 percent drop in the perception that mentally ill people are dangerous (Dunion and Gordon, 2005). A meta-analysis of public stigma-reduction interventions that included educational programs, found decreases in stigma related to mental illness, psychosis, depression, and all diagnoses combined (Griffiths et al., 2014). Notably, there was no advantage to internet-based interventions over face-to-face interventions (Griffiths et al., 2014).

See Me was a multiyear campaign delivered over multiple platforms. In contrast, a brief social media intervention in Canada called *In One Voice*[1] resulted in improved attitudes toward mental health issues and less social distance at the 1-year follow-up. However, the participants reported that they did not gain knowledge or confidence about how to help someone experiencing a mental health problem, nor did the intervention motivate young people to engage in more helpful or supportive behaviors toward those with mental health needs. The authors concluded that their study contributes to a growing body of evidence showing that

---

[1]For more information about In One Voice, see http://www.mindcheck.ca/inonevoice [March 2016].

brief media anti-stigma and mental health literacy campaigns do not result in significant and lasting change, especially in the area of behavior (Livingston et al., 2014).

A review of European anti-stigma programs found that adolescents especially showed significant change in their beliefs and attitudes in response to education (Borschmann et al., 2014). There is more variance in adolescents' beliefs about mental illness than in adults' beliefs, which may partly explain their greater responsiveness to educational interventions. Corrigan and colleagues (2012) observed that across all studies included in their meta-analysis, education was more effective than contact-base interventions in changing stigmatizing attitudes among adolescents. Adults' attitudes about mental illness and help-seeking behaviors also vary by age. In a recent national survey, younger adults were more likely than older adults to view help-seeking as a sign of strength and more likely to believe that suicide is preventable. Adults aged 54 and under were also more likely to have received treatment for a mental health condition than were those aged 55 and over (American Foundation for Suicide Prevention, 2015).

Among adolescents, online information-gathering and social support-seeking are especially popular (Birnbaum et al., 2014). When first experiencing the onset of symptoms of mental disorders, many adolescents turn to the internet as their first source of advice. In a 2014 study, Birnbaum and colleagues examined the online results yielded from hypothetical search terms used by adolescents experiencing the onset of symptoms of schizophrenia. The research team entered queries, such as "Is it normal to hear voices?" and "Do I have schizophrenia?" into Google, Facebook, and Twitter to determine the accuracy of the search results. Overwhelmingly the search results failed to direct people toward professional evaluation and some of the search results were stigmatizing in nature (Birnbaum et al., 2014).

Educational campaigns that provide information about the biogenesis of mental illness by highlighting the genetic components of schizophrenia have sometimes had unintended and stigmatizing consequences. Such messages were used to reduce the blame placed on mentally ill people for their condition (Schomerus et al., 2012). Despite their medical accuracy, these messages can intensify negative attitudes and behaviors by unintentionally drawing attention to the "differentness" of mentally ill people and diverting attention from the possibility of recovery. For example, one meta-analysis found that, when educational materials highlighted biogenetic causes of mental illness, participants were less likely to blame people with mental illness; however, they were more likely to believe that people with mental illness had low chances of recovery and more likely to say that they did not want to interact with them (Kvaale et al., 2013a). In addition, biogenetic messages may unintentionally trigger a message of hopelessness in people with mental illness, which can reinforce self-stigma and inhibit the pursuit of wellness goals (Kvaale et al., 2013a). Although these historical efforts were successful in decreasing attributional stigma, they are no longer considered effective or sufficient stigma change strategies by themselves (Corrigan et al., 2012).

Social media can also perpetuate negative stereotypes about mental and substance use disorders. In a 2015 study, Joseph and colleagues analyzed tweets about diabetes and schizophrenia, to compare the attitudes toward and perceptions of these chronic illnesses in informal online conversations. They found that tweets about schizophrenia were significantly less likely to be medically accurate and more likely to be sarcastic and negative in tone than tweets about diabetes (Joseph et al., 2015).

Mental Health Literacy Campaigns

Mental health literacy programs are a common educational strategy. Educators, health professionals, and policy makers have recognized the important role of schools in addressing the mental health needs of young people and have endorsed the implementation of school mental health programs (Wei et al., 2013). There is evidence that some in-school mental health literacy programs improve knowledge, attitudes, and help-seeking behavior, but more research is needed before decisions to scale-up mental health literacy campaigns to the national level. There is also some evidence that basic health education to improve mental health literacy may be effective in reducing stigma for school-age children; however, to improve public attitudes without negatively impacting self-stigma, the curricula need to be recovery focused and developmentally and cognitively tailored to different age groups (Wei et al., 2013). One such program is mental health first-aid, in-person training that teaches participants to respond to developing mental health problems and crises.[2]

Mental health literacy campaigns have also focused on how to encourage individuals and families to seek needed services (Jorm, 2012). This is an important goal because early diagnosis and treatment are predictive of improved outcomes, but high-quality, culturally informed treatment is not widely available, especially to racial and ethnic minority groups (Pescosolido et al., 2008a). The behavioral model of health service use, which was first used to identify factors that influenced families' utilization of health care services (Andersen, 1995), has been expanded for use in examining health-seeking behaviors for many different groups including

---

[2]For more information on mental health first aid, see http://www.mentalhealthfirstaid. org [March 2016].

minorities and children and adolescents. Eiraldi and colleagues (2006) used the original model to develop a help-seeking model for mental health service use among ethnic minority families. They identified four stages in the process of deciding to seek care for a child with symptoms of attention deficit hyperactivity disorder: problem recognition, the decision to seek help, service selection, and service utilization. The researchers noted that the problem-recognition stage is particularly important as it is the first step in access to care. Families are more likely to seek treatment for symptoms attributed to illness than for symptoms attributed to family relations or personality factors (Yeh et al., 2005).

Although campaigns that promote biogenic explanations of mental and substance use disorders are not generally effective in reducing perceptions of dangerousness and desire for social distance among the general public, there is evidence that biogenic cause attributions reduce blame (Kvaale et al., 2013a, 2013b). Biogenic explanations may help counter culturally specific negative attitudes about mental disorders (Angermeyer et al., 2011; Yang et al., 2013) and promote parental help-seeking behaviors for children's mental health problems. Efforts to close the treatment gap in access to mental health care between whites and ethnic minorities might include campaigns that target ethnic minority parents, as well as trusted community figures with messages about the biological underpinnings of mental illnesses.

Contact

Across a wide range of stigmatizing conditions, people without the stigmatized conditions have little meaningful contact with those who have these conditions. Lack of contact fosters discomfort, distrust, and fear (Cook et al., 2014). Contact interventions aim to overcome this interpersonal divide and facilitate positive interaction and connection between these groups (Shera, 1996). In contact-based behavioral health anti-stigma interventions, people with lived experience of mental illness or substance use disorders interact with the public describing their challenges and stories of success. These strategies are aimed at reducing public stigma on a person-to-person basis but have also been shown to benefit self-stigma by creating a sense of empowerment and boosting self-esteem (Corrigan et al., 2013).

Historically, contact with people with mental and substance use disorders occurred in person and through video, but now contact increasingly occurs over the internet. A Norwegian survey conducted in 2002 found that almost 75 percent of participants found it easier to discuss personal problems online rather than face to face, and almost 50 percent said they discuss problems online that they do not discuss face to face. Many comments from survey respondents demonstrated that online mental health forums have an empowering effect (Kummervold et al., 2002).

For young people in particular, online interaction might be especially beneficial and appealing. Online help-seeking is quite prevalent among adolescents who often feel empowered online and take comfort in the anonymity an online environment provides (Gould et al., 2002; Suzuki and Calzo, 2004). The Australian internet-based mental health service Reach Out! is aimed at young adults aged 16 to 25 and has been heavily trafficked (with more than 230,000 individual visits per month). Reach Out! is a safe place for young adults to seek support and share strategies and resources for dealing with mental health challenges (Webb et al., 2008).

Frequently, contact-based interventions are combined with education where factual information is presented, and the people with lived experience support and personalize the information by relating it to their own life experiences. Results of a meta-analysis of 79 studies found that effect sizes for contact on attitude change and intended behaviors were twice those of education alone (Corrigan et al., 2012). In another meta-analysis, interventions combining education and contact were equally effective as education-only interventions (Griffiths et al., 2014). Although combined interventions generally show an advantage over educational interventions alone, they are implemented less often (Borschmann et al., 2014; Corrigan et al, 2012).

A systematic review of anti-stigma programs aimed at college students by Yamaguchi and colleagues (2013) found that in-person contact and video contact were the most effective intervention types for changing attitudes and reducing social distance. Corrigan and colleagues (2012) found that in-person contact is superior to video contact, with in-person contact having twice the effect size as video contact. A systematic review of 13 studies found that education and contact-based interventions are commonly used for stigma related to substance use disorders (Livingston et al., 2012), but because of the overall dearth of studies with this focus, it is not possible to draw firm conclusions about the value of contact-based interventions over educational interventions. The preponderance of available evidence suggests that interventions that combine contact with education will be most effective.

Peer Services

Because contact-based strategies can be used to reduce both public and self-stigma, there is a wide range of potential intervention targets. One approach to integrating contact-based interventions into day-to-day activities is through the use of peer services (see Chapter 3). Peer service providers are people with lived experience who work as health care team members and foster the provision of nonjudgmental, nondiscriminatory services while openly identifying their own experiences. When integrated into service-provision teams, peers can help others to identify problems and suggest effective coping strategies (Armstrong et al., 1995; Corrigan and Phelan, 2004; Davidson et al., 1999; Gates et al., 1998; Mowbray, 1997). An example is found in Active Minds, a grassroots college student mental health advocacy group that reaches out to young people on college campuses across the United States with several programs including a speakers bureau.[3]

Peer support also acts as a counterbalance to the discrimination, rejection, and isolation people may encounter when trying to seek mental or substance use treatment and services. The supportive effects of peer interventions can help sustain longer term and more regular treatment utilization (Deegan, 1992; Markowitz, 2001; Solomon, 2004). At the same time, taking on a "helper role" can be beneficial to peer service providers on their path to recovery (Anthony, 2000; Mowbray, 1997; Schiff, 2004; Solomon, 2004). Ultimately, peer services can advance both the rights and the services agenda by facilitating treatment-seeking, fostering greater employment options, enhancing quality of life, and increasing self-efficacy in the peer service providers (Akabas and Kurzman, 2005; Gates and Akabas, 2007).

The value of peer support services in both traditional health care settings and independent programs is well recognized. In 2007, the Centers for Medicare & Medicaid issued guidelines for development and implementation of peer support services; and in 2009, the Substance Abuse and Mental Health Services Administration (SAMHSA) released the *Consumer-Operated Service Evidence-Based Practices Toolkit*.[4] Some stakeholders groups are concerned about the professionalization or medicalization of peer support services (Ostrow and Adams, 2012), while others welcome efforts to introduce uniform standards for training and practice. Professionalization of peer services can be seen as part of overall efforts to improve the quality of behavioral health care and services in the United States through a certification process, such as those that exist for other providers of care and services to those with mental and substance use disorders.

One example of these efforts at the national level is the National

---

[3]For more information on the Active Minds Speakers Bureau, see http://activeminds.org/our-programming/active-minds-speakers-bureau [March 2016].

[4]SAMHSA's Consumer-Operated Service Evidence-Based Practices Toolkit can be found at https://store.samhsa.gov/shin/content/SMA11-4633CD-DVD/TheEvidence-COSP.pdf [March 2016].

Federation of Families for Children's Mental Health's national certification program for parents who provide support services to other parents raising a child with a behavioral health disorder. The Certified Parent Support Provider™ certification defines the uniform standards and the title of parents helping other parents who have children (aged 0 to 26) experiencing emotional, behavioral health, substance or mental health disorders or intellectual disabilities. The goal of the program is to decrease the stigma associated with behavioral health disorders and promote effective strength-based children's services that are family driven and youth guided. The program has spurred the development of a peer support workforce that can be mobilized across states. A certification commission provides independent oversight to the program and has developed guidelines for achieving competency in a wide range of domains: communication, confidentiality, current issues in children's behavioral health treatment and prevention information, decision making and effecting change, educational information, empowerment, ethics, multisystem advocacy, parenting for resiliency, use of local resources, and wellness and natural support.

Protest and Advocacy

Protest strategies are rooted in advancing civil rights agendas. In the context of this report, protest is formal objection to negative representations of people with mental illness or the nature of these illnesses. Protests are often carried out at the grassroots level by those who have experienced discrimination and by advocates on their behalf. Strategies typically employ letter writing, product boycotts, or public demonstrations (Arboleda-Flórez and Stuart, 2012). Protest messaging and advocacy can help to engage and activate "fence sitters"—people who have some investment in behavioral health stigma change but limited knowledge about how to translate their beliefs into action. A call to action can also energize unengaged stakeholders by raising awareness about the harmful effects of stigma. Group protests also provide opportunities for stakeholders to meet and develop a sense of solidarity and common purpose.

Target groups for protest and advocacy campaigns are opinion leaders, such as politicians, journalists, or community officials. The goal is typically to suppress negative attitudes or to remove negative representations or content. When protest focuses on legislative reform, the goal is often to enhance or enact protections of rights, increase access to social resources, and reduce inequalities. Protest can also serve to increase public awareness and/or policy recognition of issues and concerns related to mental health (Arboleda-Flórez and Stuart, 2012).

Among the behavioral health stigma change strategies discussed in this chapter, protest is the least studied (Griffiths et al., 2014). The HIV/AIDS movement provides a model for understanding the value of protest as a stigma change strategy and underscores the importance of evaluating both intended and unintended consequences. For example, the AIDS Coalition to Unleash Power (ACT UP) began in 1987 and continued over the course of more than 2 decades. Activities in the early years of the campaign included ACT UP members chaining themselves to the offices of pharmaceutical companies involved in the development of experimental drug treatment. This tactic was widely credited with changing the way HIV/AIDS drugs were developed and delivered. In 1989, ACT UP members occupied St. Patrick's Cathedral to protest the policies of the Roman Catholic archbishop of New York, which had the unintended consequence of reframing the public debate to focus on the issue of religious freedom (DeParle, 1990).

The National Alliance on Mental Illness encourages members to become "stigma busters" and participate in such efforts. Unfortunately, the available evidence concerning the outcomes of protest related to mental illness suggests that while protest may have positive outcomes in some instances, these strategies may also trigger psychological reactance or a rebound effect in which negative public opinion is strengthened as a result of the protest (Corrigan et al., 2001). Monitoring discussions around protest and related strategies in newspapers, radio, and television, as well as social media can aid in efforts to evaluate the outcomes of these strategies. The internet serves as a potential platform for advocacy and for monitoring changes in social norms. Psychiatrists and psychologists in particular have been identified as potentially valuable voices against stigma online, and there are calls for health professionals to take up advocacy blogging to further educate the public about mental health conditions and counter stigmatizing stereotypes (Peek et al., 2015).

Legislative and Policy Change

The United States has a long history of using legal and policy interventions to protect and normalize stigmatized groups (Cook et al., 2014), significantly beginning with the Civil Rights Act of 1964, which prohibited discrimination by race, color, religion, and national origin in all public accommodations. In the 1960s and 1970s, there was a significant drop in the mortality rate of black Americans that can be linked to legislation that prohibited racial discrimination in Medicare payments for hospital-based care (Almond et al., 2006; Krieger et al., 2008).

In 2008, in part as result of mental health advocacy efforts, Congress amended the Americans with Disabilities Act (ADA) to allow people with mental illness to be covered by the ADA even when medication reduced their symptoms. Prior to the passage of the ADA Amendments Act (ADAAA), people who responded to treatment and learned to manage their symptoms lost their protections under the ADA. The ADAAA also recognizes that people may have intermittent symptoms and that some people are treated unfairly as a result of perceived rather than actual impairment. The ADAAA's attention to the specifics of functional impairment and its nuanced approach to include discrimination based on perception stands in contrast to legislation that applies more arbitrary inclusion criteria across diverse mental illnesses (Corrigan et al., 2005b).

Throughout this report, the committee stresses the important of addressing stigma at the structural level. Much of the knowledge base concerning structural stigma, including empirical evidence, concepts, and theories, comes from research on gender and ethnic or minority differences. Structural stigma can be intentional or unintentional, overt or covert. Policies that disqualify people with mental illness from receiving health insurance coverage are an example of overt structural stigma; in contract, failure of police officials to distinguish between mental health apprehensions and suicide attempts on criminal record checks is an example of covert structural stigma or of stigma at the structural level (Mental Health Commission of Canada, 2013).

Researchers in the United States have found that people with mental illness favor approaches that address institutional and structural discrimination over those that focus on public education (Mental Health Commission of Canada, 2013). In a U.S. survey of individuals with psychiatric disabilities, one-quarter to one-half of respondents reported the experience of discrimination in social arenas, including employment (52%), housing (32%), law enforcement (27%), and education (24%) (Corrigan et al., 2003). Addressing sources of structural stigma can also promote mental and physical well-being, for example, medical and mental health care visits by lesbians, gay men, and bisexuals decreased after same-sex marriage was legalized in Massachusetts (Hatzenbuehler et al., 2012), and depression and anxiety in members of low-income families decreased when the families were provided with rental vouchers (Anderson et al., 2003).

Multidisciplinary, multilevel ecological approaches are needed to understand and address structural stigma and to engage groups and organizations, including lawyers, journalists, educators, and business and property owners, to address the root causes of structural stigma. Stigma researchers and mental health advocates suggest that anti-stigma efforts should not focus narrowly on "soft goals" of public education and attitude change but should expand their focus to address "hard goals," such as legislative and policy change that can promote social equity and improve overall quality of life for people with mental and substance use disorders (Mental Health Commission of Canada, 2013; Stuart et al., 2012; Thornicroft et al., 2007).

EVIDENCE FROM LARGE-SCALE CAMPAIGNS

The section describes the findings from large-scale campaigns in and outside the United States, including three national-level campaigns from Australia (beyondblue), Canada (Opening Minds), and England (Time to Change). The large-scale campaigns in the United States reviewed by the committee included the Eliminations of Barriers Initiative and What a Difference a Friend Makes, along with notable state-based initiatives such as the California Mental Health Services Authority, and efforts on the part of the U.S. Departments of Defense and Veterans Affairs (VA) to reduce mental health stigma and encourage treatment-seeking among members of the military and military veterans, including Make the Connection and the Real Warriors campaign.

Under the California Mental Health Services Act, a statewide prevention and early intervention program was set up, composed of three strategic initiatives that focused on (1) reduction of stigma and discrimination toward those with mental illness, (2) prevention of suicide, and (3) improvement in student mental health. Each initiative is implemented with the help of community partner agencies. Preliminary evaluations of the act show that social marketing materials designed for the program reached a large number of Californians. Beyond the reach of the materials, findings show that stigma against mental illness has decreased in California, with more people reporting a willingness to socialize with, live next door to, and work with people experiencing mental illness. People also reported that they are providing greater social support to those with mental illness (Collins et al., 2015).

The VA's Make the Connection website hosts a wealth of behavioral health resources for veterans, and serves as a venue by which veterans can share their lived experiences. In particular, Make the Connection focuses on sharing positive stories of veterans who reached out to receive help for their mental health problems (Langford et al., 2013).

The Real Warriors campaign is a large-scale multimedia program with the goal of facilitating recovery, promoting resilience, and supporting the reintegration of service members, veterans, and families. The Real Warriors campaign is based on the health-belief model and serves as an example of an evidence-based media campaign, and notably one informed by ongoing independent evaluations (Acosta et al., 2012; Langford et al., 2013).

Large-scale anti-stigma campaigns have been undertaken in many other countries as well, for example, Scotland's See Me campaign,[5] a long-term effort begun in 2002 that mobilizes people and groups to work collaboratively with a focus on negative behavior change and human rights issues; One of Us,[6] a relatively new (2011) campaign in Denmark that includes a focus on young people, the labor market, service uses and providers, and the media; and Spain's 1decada4 campaign,[7] which seeks to make mental illness more visible to increase social acceptance of the one in four people who will have a mental disorder during their lives.

The committee focused on Time to Change (England), Opening Minds (Canada), and beyondblue (Australia) because of the national-level scale of these campaigns and the robustness of the outcome evaluations (see Table 4-1). The committee invited researchers from these three campaigns to present their findings at a public workshop held by the committee in April 2015 (see Appendix A).

Presenters were asked to address three questions: (1) What did they do? (2) How did they evaluate the campaign? and (3) What did they find? The researchers were also asked to share both the successes and the challenges of the campaigns. The committee members discussed the information obtained during the workshops and from the relevant peer-reviewed literature and deliberated about how best to apply the findings within a U.S. context. The three foreign campaigns are summarized below based on the key questions stated above. The information presented in these summaries was drawn from the researchers' presentations, published reports of campaign outcomes, and the peer-reviewed literature.

Table 4-1 and the discussion that follows summarize the lessons learned from successful well-evaluated national-scale campaigns about how to inform a national dialogue and improve public attitudes and behaviors concerning people with mental and substance use disorders at the population level using multifaceted, long-term strategies that engage state, local, and grassroots community groups; permit the scaling up of successful smaller scale interventions; and facilitate research on what works to reduce stigma in population subgroups, such as racial and ethnic minorities and relevant target groups, such as educators, employers, and health care providers.

---

[5]For more Information about Scotland's See Me campaign, see https://www.seeme scotland.org/ [March 2016].

[6]For more information about Denmark's One of Us, see the campaign's English-language website at http://www.en-af-os.dk/English.aspx/ [March 2016].

[7]For more information about Spain's 1decada4, see the campaign's English-language website at http://www.1decada4.es/course/view.php?id=2 [March 2016].

TABLE 4-1 National Campaigns Modeling Successful Interventions

Title of Campaign/ Country	Intervention Components	Time Frame	Cost
Time to Change (England)	▪ Social marketing and mass media activity ▪ Local community events to bring people with and without mental health problems together ▪ A grant scheme to fund grassroots projects led by people with mental health problems ▪ A program to empower a network of people with experience of mental health problems to challenge discrimination ▪ Targeted work with stakeholders to improve practice and policy ▪ Research and evaluation	2008-2015 (ongoing)	$60 million thru 2015/£40 million
Opening Minds (Canada)	▪ Grassroots contact-based education programs aimed at o youths aged 12-18 o health care providers o employers and the workforce o news media o research and evaluation	2009-2015 (ongoing)	$2 million annually, ($14 million to date)
beyondblue (Australia)	▪ Mass-media advertising ▪ Community education programs ▪ Training of prominent people as champions ▪ Digital and print materials ▪ Mental health literacy ▪ Community discussion forums ▪ Mindframe, a national media initiative about responsible reporting of suicide ▪ Research and evaluation	2000-2015 (ongoing)	$38 million from 2000-2005; $80 million from 2005-2010

Time to Change

Findings from the evaluation of Time to Change in England highlight the importance of long-term data collection, establishment of baseline trends, and ensuring a match between complex, evolving social processes such as prejudice and acceptance with nuanced (triangulated) evaluation methods, while specifying outcome indicators (targets for change) as knowledge, attitudes, or behaviors (Evans-Lacko et al., 2013a).

What Did They Do?

Time to Change is England's largest ever program to reduce stigma and discrimination against people with mental health problems.[8] The project began in 2008 and is ongoing. Funding covered the development and implementation of the anti-stigma activities, as well as evaluation activities, including the collection of nationally representative baseline data and follow-on surveys of the English population from which progress could be measured in the future. Between 2008 and 2015, the project received £40 million ($60 million U.S.) to design and deliver a multiphase, multifaceted campaign that included

- social marketing and mass media activity at the national level to raise awareness of mental health issues;
- local community events to bring people with and without mental health problems together;
- a grant program to fund grassroots projects led by people with mental health problems;
- a program to empower a network of people with experience of mental health problems to challenge discrimination; and
- targeted work with stakeholders, for example, medical students, teachers in training, employers, and young people.

Funding also allowed the campaign to do formative research during the first year involving more than 4,000 people with direct experience of mental health problems to provide input on stigma and discrimination and specific targets for change, which then guided the campaign.

---

[8]For more information about England's Time to Change, see http://www.time-to-change.org/uk [March 2016].

Examples of Activities

Based on insight from the developmental phase, the mass media campaign (including national television, print, radio, and outdoor and online advertisement and social media as well as cinema) targeted specific groups of individuals. The film Schizo,[9] one component of the national-level campaign, was shown in movie theatres across the country, and later adapted for use in the United States. Nationally representative surveys of the general public concerning knowledge, attitudes, and behavior in relation to people with mental health problems were used to assess change over time. At the community and grassroots levels, the project included varied activities based on the theme "start a conversation." Community-level social contact included "Living Libraries" where, instead of borrowing only books, library visitors could borrow a person and hear about firsthand experiences of stigma discrimination from those with lived experience of mental illness. Data were collected at the community level during these social contact events in different cities across England to assess the relationship between the quality of the social contact and intended stigmatizing behavior and campaign engagement. Grassroots-level components also included volunteer-led activities (contact-based and peer-service programs) at college campuses and other public places that provided data on the impact of disclosure of mental or substance use disorders on self-stigma and the sense of well-being and empowerment, again through the use of validated tools.

How Did They Evaluate the Campaign?

Time to Change is notable for the depth and breadth of its evaluation. Although the campaign included various types of activities at multiple levels of society, the main outcome measures were common across most activities. To assess changes among the general public, the main outcome measures included the following validated assessments: (1) change in knowledge measured by the 12- item Mental Health Knowledge Schedule) comprising 6 items to assess stigma-related mental health knowledge and 6 items about the classification of conditions as a mental illness; (2) change in attitudes using 26-item Community Attitudes Toward Mental Illness, covering attitudes related to prejudice and exclusion and also tolerance and support for community care; and (3) change in behavior, both reported and intended, assessed using the 8-item Reported and Intended

---

[9]The film can be viewed on YouTube, see https://www.youtube.com/watch?v=J-JV-BO7nLv0 [March 2016].

Behavior Scale (RIBS).[10] Additionally, 1,000 people with a diagnosed mental illness and recently in contact with secondary mental health services were interviewed annually (different individuals each year) about the discrimination they face using the Discrimination and Stigma Scale. Additional assessments included monitoring of changes in media reporting; surveys of relevant groups including trainee teachers, medical students, and employers; and cost-benefit analyses.

What Did They Find?

The multilevel, multifaceted approach increased public understanding of stigma and discrimination against people with mental illness, which formative research in the first year had revealed to be low at the start of the project. Triangulation, use of a variety of different research methods, allowed the researchers to tease apart complex social norms about mental illness and increased understanding of the mediating role of social contact in explaining the effects of the anti-stigma interventions. The findings also underscore the importance of measuring both direct and indirect effects, and to consider the mechanisms of change including openness and disclosure, contact, and awareness.

The national scale social marketing campaign included mass media components and assessment of knowledge, attitudes, and behavior across the country. The social marketing mass media component of the campaign was most effective at influencing intended behavior toward people with mental illness. Despite a lack of improvement overall in knowledge or attitudes, one RIBS survey item ("In the future, I would be willing to live with someone with a mental health problem") showed consistent improvement (from 29.3 to 44.4%) across the total target population. Other intended behaviors, including willingness to work with, live nearby, or continue a relationship with someone with a mental health problem, showed more modest improvements. Critically, there was also a significant reduction in levels of discrimination reported by people with mental illness. Assessment of newspaper coverage across England revealed an increased proportion of balanced, anti-stigmatizing articles reporting on mental health issues.

Time to Change adds to the growing evidence base supporting the effectiveness of social contact and demonstrates the value of creativity in designing community level, contact-based programs to reduce public stigma. The grassroots-level activities reduced self-stigma through its community initiatives. Among the participants with mental health prob-

---

[10] For further information on the validated scales, see http://www.kcl.ac.uk/ioppn/depts/hspr/research/ciemh/cmh/CMH-Measures.aspx [March 2016].

lems, almost one-half (49%) reported that they had disclosed their condition during the event. A similar proportion of participants (48%) said that they had met someone with a mental health problem during the event, and more than half of all participants (58%) said they had met someone without a mental health problem during the event. These outcomes are salient because selective disclosure can facilitate positive social contact, and intergroup interactions between people with and without mental illness helps reduce stigmatizing "us versus them" thinking.

Participants were asked to describe their meetings in terms of positive contact factors including the sense of social equity and the feeling of working together toward common goals. People without mental illness who reported more contact factors were more likely to say that they would be more supportive of people with mental illness in the future (Evans-Lacko et al., 2012b). In this study, data were synthesized from a number of interventions across England. The findings indicate that social contact interventions can be implemented and evaluated on a large scale, and suggest that larger sample sizes and the use of control groups could facilitate research on differences among population subgroups.

Finally, Time to Change provides data on the cost-effectiveness of long-term, multilevel, national-scale anti-stigma efforts. Phase one of the campaign was rolled out in six successive "bursts" with public awareness of the campaign measured after each burst ("Can you think of any campaigns, that is advertising or events in the local community, you have seen or heard concerning mental health or mental health problems?"). Awareness was strongly associated with campaign burst expenditure and increased awareness was positively associated with increased knowledge, more favorable attitudes, and improved intended behavior. Project estimates of the cost of improved intended behavior toward people with mental illness range from £2 to £4 ($3-$6) per person. The annual program cost for Time to Change was 0.01 percent of the annual cost of mental health care in the United Kingdom, less than the amounts spent for analogous public health campaigns on obesity (0.12%), alcohol misuse (0.04%), and stroke (0.18%).

beyondblue

In the 1990s, the Australian government launched a national initiative to improve the knowledge and skills of primary care practitioners and other health professionals regarding mental health problems. At the time, the knowledge and skills of the general public were not seen as important. To draw attention to this gap, the researchers coined the term "mental health literacy," defined as "knowledge and beliefs about mental disorders that aid their recognition, management, or prevention." They defined the components of mental health literacy as:

- recognition of the disorders in oneself and others to facilitate help-seeking,
- knowledge of professional help and treatment availability,
- knowledge of effective self-help strategies,
- knowledge and skills to provide aid and support to others, and
- knowledge about how to prevent mental disorders.

What Did They Do?

beyondblue is an Australian not-for-profit organization that began as "beyondblue: the national depression initiative" but now addresses both depression and anxiety. The initiative grew out of efforts beginning in the 1990s to improve the knowledge and skills of primary care practitioners to address mental health problems. The goal of the mental health literacy campaign was to raise awareness of the importance of the public's knowledge, beliefs, and skills related to mental disorders, including prevention and treatment. There were five priority areas: community awareness and de-stigmatization, consumer and caregiver support, prevention and early intervention, primary care training and support, and applied research. Information was disseminated and messages conveyed over multiple media platforms, including television, radio, the internet, and print media. beyondblue partnered with an organization called Schools Television to raise awareness and provide information about mental illness and engaged well-known actors to talk openly about their personal experiences with mental illness (Dunt et al., 2010).

The activities are largely funded by the Australian national government and some of the territorial (state) governments, with some financial and in-kind support from nongovernmental sources. The organization began its work in 2000 as a 5-year initiative yet it continues.

Examples of Activities

There were many varied activities including mass-media advertising, sponsorship of events, community education programs, training of prominent people as champions, and web and print information. Mental Health First Aid training was developed in Australia in 2000 by Betty Kitchener starting as a small volunteer effort that has now been replicated in many other countries (Clay, 2013). Other prominent interventions included Mind Matters, programs in high school that are incorporated into regular lessons; RUOK Day—people ask others about their mental well-being "Are you OK?"; Rotary community forums on mental illness across the country that involve elected officials and average citizens; and Mindframe, a national media initiative that includes training programs and guidelines for responsible reporting about suicide. The campaign also provides funding to initiate and continue research on depression and anxiety, and over the course of the campaign, the funded research activities have grown in number and been more aligned with stakeholder-identified priorities (Dunt et al., 2010).

What Did They Find?

Periodic surveys of national mental health literacy were conducted in Australia from the mid-1990s allowing researchers to monitor trends in public attitudes before and during the implementation of beyondblue. Survey respondents viewed vignettes of depressed persons and then responded to questions about a range of possible interventions (seeing a psychologist, taking antidepressants, having psychotherapy, and dealing with it alone) and whether they thought these would be effective in treating depression. During its first 5 years, beyondblue had higher levels of activity in some Australian states and territories than in others, creating de facto treatment and control groups. In states with higher levels of activities (those that provided a higher level of support), there was greater improvement in public awareness of depression as a problem, beliefs about the benefits and efficacy of treatment, and positive attitudes about people with depression (Jorm, 2012; Jorm et al., 2005, 2006).

Meta-analyses of trials of Mental Health First Aid training program outcomes show moderate increases in knowledge about mental illness and smaller effects on attitudes and behaviors. Improvements were sustained over 6 months. To date, the program has trained and certified 2 percent of Australian adults, with a goal of 11 percent. People and organizations will pay for this training as they pay for other first-aid training. This allows program sustainability beyond government funding periods (Jorm and Kitchener, 2011).

Although the researchers are not certain which interventions led to these improvements, it is clear that the concept of mental health literacy as a desirable aim was incorporated into national and state policy goals. A national survey found that at the 10-year mark in the implementation of the campaign 87 percent of Australians were aware of its work. Between the publication of the first beyondblue report in 2004 and the second in 2009, there was a significant nationwide increase in the availability of primary care services for depression (Dunt et al., 2010). According to the 2009 report, researchers were unable to determine whether people with depression experienced a reduction in stigma and discrimination as public awareness increased, and although survey data show a steady decrease in social distance overtime. Public perception of depressed people as dangerous (68%) and unpredictable (52%) persists.

Opening Minds

The Mental Health Commission of Canada was launched in 2007 with federal funding. Opening Minds is the ongoing anti-stigma initiative of the commission and was launched in 2009 with a 10-year mandate and an annual budget of $2 million.[11] Its goal is to change the attitudes and behaviors of Canadians toward people with a mental illness and to encourage individuals, groups, and organizations to eliminate discrimination. It is the largest systematic effort of its kind in the history of Canada. In February 2015, the Opening Minds initiative won the global innovator award at the Together Against Stigma International Conference in San Francisco, California.

What Did They Do?

The commission began Opening Minds with a small, public education media campaign designed to communicate positive messages about people with mental illness. The results were disappointing and the commission decided against a costly, long-term social media campaign (Stuart et al., 2014b).

Instead, the project team issued a request for interest. It was distributed to a wide network of government agencies, universities, stakeholders, and existing grassroots anti-stigma programs across Canada. These initiatives shared one thing in common: they all used some form of contact-based education. The project team linked them with Opening Minds researchers for evaluation and scale-up of effective programs. Work focused on four target groups: youths aged 12-18, health care providers, the workforce or employers, and the news media. Principal investigators were recruited from leading Canadian universities for each target group.

The project teams used similar evaluation strategies so that researchers could compare outcomes across settings to help determine which program activities would yield the greatest effects. The goal was to develop effective, evidence-based models that could be replicated and disseminated to other communities and stakeholders who want to begin anti-stigma efforts.

---

[11]See http://www.mentalhealthcommission.ca/English/initiatives-and-projects/opening-minds [March 2016].

Examples of Activities

One activity is "HEADSTRONG," a program targeting youth. This activity brings together youth from local high schools to a regional summit where they participate in exercises, learn about the problems created by stigma, and hear stories from people with lived experience of mental health problems or mental illnesses. Equipped with toolkits and examples of anti-stigma activities, these students go back to their schools and lead anti-stigma efforts bringing mental health awareness along with messages of hope and recovery. The youth champions are also supported by a coordinator who links them with a coalition of community groups, which also provides resources and access to speakers.

HEADSTRONG included and involved

- 19 regional coordinators,
- 132 students at a National Summit,
- 27 regional summits in the 2014-2015 school year,
- 3 provincial events with HEADSTRONG activities and workshops, and
- approximately 4,450 student participants (with the potential to reach approximately 186,000 high school students through future school-based activities and community coalitions).

Another activity was "Understanding Stigma", an anti-stigma program aimed at health care professionals that emerged as one of Opening Mind's most effective anti-stigma programs. The program comprises a 2-hour workshop that includes six key ingredients such as a Power-Point show of famous people with mental illness that also functions as an introduction to stigma; a group exercise comparing earaches with depression to illustrate the need for timely treatment and social support; a short discussion of the definition of stigma as a form of prejudice and discrimination; along with locally made films, myth-busting (countering myths about mental illness), and a keynote speech by a person with mental illness that engenders discussion among participants. Workshops were originally developed for use by emergency room staff, but they were later adapted for other groups. The program objectives are to raise awareness among health professionals of their own attitudes; to provide them with an opportunity to hear personal stories of mental illness, hope, and recovery from people with mental illness; and to demonstrate that health care providers can make a positive difference. The program also includes pre- and posttests as well as take-home resources and the opportunity to sign an anti-stigma commitment.

Opening Minds has also produced a guide for media reporting on mental health. *Mindset: Reporting on Mental Health*[12] includes sections that help journalists distinguish among various mental disorders (stressing that mental illness is a broad category and reporting should specify diagnoses), and guidelines for interviewing people with and about mental illness, and appropriate language to use when reporting on mental illness, suicide, and addiction.

How Did They Evaluate the Campaign?

Researchers evaluated the Opening Minds programs using mixed methods, including qualitative methods such as focus groups and standardized instruments to measure stigma and social distance pre- and postprogram implementation. The researchers developed fidelity scales for contact-based education programs. This was done to ensure that programs followed best practice guidelines.

What Did They Find?

In the Opening Minds campaign, researchers worked with existing anti-stigma initiatives and aided them in evaluating their programs and implementing change to improve those outcomes. This approach allowed the team to develop a set of evidence-based criteria for evaluating programs. Among the findings documented in the interim report on Opening Mind's (2013) are that some programs for young people actually did harm by concretizing negative stereotypes. Similarly, while contact-based education programs were the most effective type of anti-stigma effort overall, the message matters and the most successful programs featured stories of hope and recovery. Finally, peer training and support was essential as storytellers had to be psychologically ready to share their stories, able to engage the audience, and handle questions and open discussions.

Design and delivery were important factors in the success of the programs for health professionals, but short programs worked as well as longer programs. The most successful programs used multiple forms of contact-based education, including live personal testimony as well as taped events. Successful programs had incentives or expectations of participation by the health care professionals, such as continuing education credits, being paid for their time, or receiving paid time off. Physicians were particularly difficult to engage. In a meta-analysis of the findings from more than 20 "Understanding Stigma" programs aimed at health professionals, the researchers found that the quality of the contact pro-

---

[12]For more information about the Mindset Media Guide, see http://www.mindset-media guide.ca/ [March 2016].

vided was more important than the duration of the contact, and that the interventions that included all six key ingredients had the strongest positive outcomes. The ingredients most predictive of positive change were messages that focused on recovery and inclusion in multiple forms or points of contact (Knaak et al., 2014).

Among the lessons learned was that programs that targeted a specific mental illness may reduce stigma to a greater degree than those that target mental illness in general. In the future, the Opening Mind's team will focus on identifying the components of successful programs, how success in reducing stigma varies by health care professional target audience, and what processes actually bring about positive changes in attitudes and intended behavior toward people with mental illness.

In an analysis of more than 20,000 print articles from 2005 to the present in Canadian newspapers along with 1,300 television reports, the campaign found that 40 percent of newspaper articles focused on crime and violence and only 20 percent focused on recovery, shortage of resources, and issues related to treatment. Less than 25 percent of the articles included the voice of someone with lived experience of mental illness or the voice of a mental health expert. As in other countries, including the United States, journalists quickly assigned psychiatric labels to people who had committed shocking crimes without solid evidence that the person had a mental illness. To change this harmful practice, Opening Minds joined with journalism schools across Canada to develop a curriculum that included contact-based education, preferably delivered by a graduate of the school. The curriculum includes the *Mindset* guide about reporting on tragic events. 5000 copies have been distributed.

The following is a summary of the findings of the Opening Minds campaign (Mental Health Commission of Canada, 2013):

- Big media campaigns are not effective at changing attitudes.
- One-time only sessions do not work, boosters are needed (immunization model).
- Voluntary attendance is not effective.
- Not all contact-based education is effective.
- Grassroots networks and local champions are needed.

Contact-based education emerged as the choice strategy for stigma reduction. Building partnerships with community and grassroots groups coupled with the development of a process for systematic evaluation and standardized interventions and outcome measures allowed the team to develop a set of best practices. The plan for the next phase is to scale-up successful approaches for nationwide implementation (Stuart et al., 2014b).

Challenges and Limitations

Evaluating large-scale, multi-intervention, multilocale, long-term initiatives is challenging. Design, methods, and measurement issues are among the major challenges, specifically, reliance on nonrandomized designs; outcome data and measurements focused on change in attitude but not change in behavior; failure to differentiate attitudes toward specific behavioral health disorders; reliance on self-report data that could have social desirability effects; absence of needed baseline data and outcome measures that change over time making longitudinal assessments difficult; and suboptimal frequency of data collection. A meta-review of media campaigns in particular found that evaluations often fail to include data on financial costs, adverse effects, and unintended consequences (Clement et al., 2013).

Limitations more specific to the large-scale initiatives described above pertained to differences in surveys for different interventions and target groups; reliance on aggregated outcome data that did not always capture small changes at the community level especially since the intensity of local initiatives varied across communities; differences in baselines across communities; and challenges in measuring the outcomes of structural interventions, such as changes in government policy and regulation as a result of initiatives. It was also difficult, given the available data, to evaluate the differential impact of the initiatives on racial and ethnic minorities and to gather data on the sustainability of the intervention outcomes (Dunt et al., 2010; Evans-Lacko et al., 2014; Jorm et al., 2005; Stuart et al., 2014a, 2014b).

5

Research Strategies

This chapter focuses on components of a research strategy that are essential to the design and evaluation of stigma reduction interventions and approaches: (1) *formative research* to assist in developing interventions and tailoring them for target audiences, (2) *intervention research* to assess implementation and outcomes of the specific interventions, and (3) *monitoring trends* over time in attitudes, beliefs, knowledge, and behaviors toward people with behavioral disorders as manifested at structural, public, and individual levels. The chapter concludes with suggested areas for future research and evaluation.

FORMATIVE RESEARCH

Launching a large-scale stigma change strategy can imbue an organization with a sense of urgency and excitement. Yet, charging forward hastily can waste resources and produce disappointing results. For a campaign to be effective and relevant to stakeholders, interventions must be well-designed and correctly targeted based on prior formative research and ongoing evaluation. Research and interventions must work in tandem and learn from one another. Formative research may also reveal new features of stigma, generate research questions, and contribute to the development of evidence-based interventions. In addition, researchers should examine naturally occurring phenomena (e.g., media events, and policy implementations) and their effect on levels of stigma as insights from these naturally occurring phenomena could inform future research, interventions, and policy initiatives.

Formative research draws from a mix of scientific disciplines, including psychology, anthropology, and sociology, and is used to design campaigns that are geographically and culturally appropriate (Gittelsohn et al., 2006). Behavior is shaped by a range of social, psychological, and structural factors making behavior change difficult to achieve. Through formative research, strategy designers define and assess the characteristics of the target audience relevant to the behavioral health issues of interest (Gittelsohn et al., 2006). The ultimate goal of formative research in this area is to identify factors, including motivating factors that can increase the effectiveness of behavioral interventions.

Community-Based Participatory Research

Beyond conducting an assessment of the potential audience, formative research is a way to facilitate relationships between the researchers and their intended audience. Incorporating formative research in the design phase of a multicomponent national strategy can ensure that the strategy is targeted to the most appropriate populations or subgroups; and that the voices of stakeholders, particularly those with lived experience, are included in the planning and evaluation of the interventions. Formative research methods that engage communities in developing initiatives include community-based participatory research, empowerment evaluation, and participatory or community action research (Ahmed and Palermo, 2010).

Participatory approaches involve and actively engage critical stakeholders (e. g., peer experts, family members, advocates, health care practitioners, provider organizations, employers, policy makers) at every stage of the research process. Stakeholders are included as active partners in understanding the problem, describing possible approaches and interventions, describing the theory of change behind interventions, identifying methods and measures to test the approach, collecting and analyzing the data that emerge from the design, and making sense of the findings (Corrigan and Shapiro, 2010). These methods are well suited to stigma change efforts because they can provide input on the subtle and dynamic aspects of stigma and discrimination that must be translated into specific interventions and messages to increase their relevance to both those who stigmatize and those who experience stigma (Corrigan and Shapiro, 2010).

Community participatory methods are useful as a component of formative research in understanding the perspectives of specific target audiences and in determining the best mechanisms or platforms to reach them. For example, attention deficit hyperactivity disorder (ADHD) is among the most common childhood mental illnesses and evidence-based psychosocial and pharmacological treatments are available. But white children are twice more likely to be assessed, diagnosed, and treated for the disorder than ethnic minority children. Although access to quality care is certainly determined by social and economic factors, a family's decision to seek mental health treatments is strongly influenced by knowledge and beliefs about mental illness. In a sample of Latino families, after controlling for socioeconomic status, family cultural values and beliefs including those about gender roles and natural or spiritual harmony/disharmony predicted attitudes about ADHD as an illness as well as attitudes about child behaviors associated with inattention or hyperactivity (Lawton and Gerdes, 2014) .

Principles of Local Tailoring

Communications research and strategies in public health should focus simultaneously on individuals, their social networks, larger communities, and the locales that influence behavior and health (Abroms and Maibach, 2008). For example, a study of the factors that led to an increase in the number of cases of autism diagnosed in California concluded that neighborhood parks, stores, and schools were places of key social interaction and information diffusion about the condition among parents. One way to understand what influences local communities and to tailor research and interventions to local areas is to involve local opinion leaders in the design and evaluation of interventions. In keeping with a "grassroots" approach to designing their national stigma reduction initiative, "Opening Minds," the Mental Health Commission of Canada evaluated the outcomes of many local initiatives and invested in scaling-up and replicating those that demonstrated effectiveness (Pietrus, 2013).

INTERVENTION RESEARCH

A strong intervention research component needs to be included in a multipronged national strategy to ensure that the various interventions (e.g., contact-based programs, educational programs, and mass media campaigns) are working as intended, and that they are producing the intended effects. The focus in this section is on measurement of stigma-related constructs, design considerations, and appropriate cost-benefit analyses.

Measurement of Stigma-Related Constructs

In line with the research on how stigma is defined and manifested, as discussed in Chapters 1 and 2, various domains are used to measure components of stigma. Most commonly measured domains include labeling, stereotyping, cognitive separating (i.e., us versus them), emotional reactions of the stigmatizer or of people who are stigmatized, interpersonal discrimination (i.e., expected, believed, or experienced), and structural discrimination (Link et al., 2004). In addition, three types of behavior are commonly measured: the behavior of people who have a mental illness that may serve as a stimulus to stigma, the behavior of people with mental illness in response to discrimination (e.g., avoidance or coping) (Link et al., 2004); and the behavior of people or institutions that are stigmatizing (e.g., discriminating, coercing, segregating) (Corrigan and Shapiro, 2010).

A review of measures used in mental illness stigma research that was conducted for the committee (Yang and Link, 2015) showed that prominent measures used to assess stigma among adult general community members cover most of the domains described above and include assessments of social distance, opinions about mental illness, community attitudes toward mental illness, semantic differential, attribution measures, emotional responses, and perceived devaluation-discrimination. The measures are established in their use and demonstrate good reliability and construct validity. In particular, the social distance, semantic differential, and opinion scales have a long history of use, and social distance and semantic differential scales have been used as the primary outcome in nationally representative surveys of attitudes toward people with mental illness in Australia (Reavley and Jorm, 2011) and the United States (see Pescosolido, 2015, for detail on concepts and measures; Pescosolido et al., 2010).

Program evaluators assessing outcomes of addictions stigma change efforts often rely on measures that have been adapted or developed specifically for studies about substance use (Pearson, 2015). Examples of mental health methods that have been adapted for use with substance use disorders include the Perceived Stigma of Addiction Scale (PSAS) to assess perceived public stigma in individuals in treatment for substance use problems (Luoma et al., 2010). The PSAS was found to be moderately correlated with measures of self-stigma including internalized shame and internalized stigma. In developing scales specific to stigma toward illicit drug use (Stigma of Drug Users Scale and the Drug Use Stigmatization Scale), Palamar and colleagues (2011) found that the two scales were measuring distinct forms of stigma: perceived (i.e., indirectly rating what most peoples' attitudes are) and stigmatization (i.e., directly rating one's own attitude). The authors also reported finding construct validity through correlations showing that higher levels of stigmatization or greater perceived public stigma were inversely related to exposure to problem users. For assessing self-stigma, the Substance Abuse Self-Stigma Scale (Luoma et al., 2013) has four subscales, based on relational frame theory, with two subscales assessing self-stigma directly (self-devaluation, fear of enacted stigma) and two subscales assessing maladaptive reactions to self-stigma (stigma avoidance, values disengagement). The scales have shown theoretically consistent associations across a range of stigma-related constructs in residential or outpatient treatment populations (Brown et al., 2015; Luoma et al., 2013).

General versus Specific Measures

Concerns arise from scales that use "mental illness" as the referent in questions. In these cases there is no way to ascertain what respondents are thinking about (e.g., schizophrenia, depression, or attention deficit hyperactivity disorder). This becomes especially problematic as research has documented very different levels of prejudice toward individuals with different mental illness and substance use disorders (Barry et al., 2014; Martin et al., 2000).

Labeled versus Case-Based Approaches

Concerns also arise from asking about a category of mental illness or substance use disorder rather than a case description. While a category provides a clear referent, it does not match what individuals observe in the real world in terms of an individual behaving in a particular manner. Further, providing a categorical label does not allow researchers to ascertain whether individuals recognize a given condition.

Construct Validity

Construct validity is the extent to which a scale or test is actually measuring what it intends to measure. This is important in stigma research at all stages from planning to evaluation because of the many perspectives and constructs that underlie the phenomenon. For example, an instrument or scale may be intended to measure public, self, or structural stigma; perceived attitudes of other people or one's own attitudes; or discrimination that is experienced or anticipated. Findings related to construct validity in stigma research are mixed. While evidence of construct validity has been found in some measures that assess public attitudes and emotions (Link et al., 2004), a recent meta-analysis (Stevelink et al., 2012) found that only one out of six mental illness-related stigma scales reviewed had acceptable construct validity. This suggests that, when selecting measures of stigma and reviewing their psychometric properties, particular attention should be paid to tests of their construct validity and the extent to which the constructs being measured correlate with other similar measures.

Social Validity

When designing programs to change behavior, it is important to ensure that the intervention is considered socially important, ethical, and acceptable to both the target of the intervention and outside observers. Social validity (sometimes referred to as ecological validity or cultural validity) is a multidimensional concept that traditionally serves as an assessment of both the *importance* of a behavioral intervention and the *acceptability* of the intervention. It is often assessed across three factors: the goals of the intervention, the intervention procedures, and the intervention outcomes (Foster and Mash, 1999). Although the discussion of how best to assess social validity is evolving, historically researchers rely on normative comparisons to assess the importance of an intervention and subjective evaluations to assess the acceptability of the intervention (Foster and Mash, 1999). Because social validity is unique to each intervention, it is critical to involve stakeholders (e.g., people with serious mental illnesses, employers, family members, providers) in formative research during the evaluation planning stages to appropriately assess the social validity of the planned intervention (Corrigan and Shapiro, 2010).

Research Methods and Design Considerations

In developing methods to evaluate specific interventions in a national anti-stigma initiative, the type of intervention and subject matter require special attention. This section briefly covers designs for evaluating the effectiveness of interventions and issues that could affect the research designs, including social desirability, external validity, and fidelity or internal validity.

Research Designs

Research designs used for evaluating the effectiveness of stigma reduction interventions are the same as those used in other social and behavioral sciences. Randomized controlled trials are considered to be the gold standard because random assignment of participants to the intervention being implemented versus a control group or comparison group allows for a causal inference to be drawn between the intervention and the outcome (Shadish et al., 2002). Randomized controlled trials are useful for everything from laboratory tests of the effectiveness of specific content and methods of persuasion to field tests of entire programs. However, randomized controlled trials are rarely used in evaluating large media campaigns because of the difficulties in random assignment and controlling conditions at community or larger scale levels (Hornik, 2002; Noar, 2006). It is also difficult to identify a comparison group that was not exposed to the campaign's message (Hornik, 2002). Time-series designs that assess processes and outcomes of campaigns at multiple points can be useful in comparing expected and actual trends in stigma and discrimination reduction (Collins et al., 2012). Alternatively, a dose-response test can be used to measure the effect of a campaign's message across different communities with different levels of exposure (Collins et al., 2012).

Social Desirability

In research studies assessing stigma, social desirability can interfere if respondents want to offer a positive image of themselves rather than respond with their truest attitude (Tourangeau and Yan, 2007). This can introduce bias in measures, and it can also pose problems in research designs that include pre- and posttest assessment or repeated measure designs when study participants may anticipate the desired response (Corrigan and Shapiro, 2010). A recent study found that "differences" (i.e., between a survey respondent and a person with mental illness) are more likely to be endorsed than "stereotypes" because differences may be considered neutral, while stereotypes are generally perceived to be negative (Corrigan et al., 2015b). Therefore, using measures of difference and incorporating repeated measures in the design may yield more sensitive indicators of stigma change.

Fidelity of an Intervention and Internal Validity

Internal validity is the degree to which researchers can conclude that findings are due to deliberate experimental manipulation rather than unaccounted for or confounding variables. Closely related, intervention fidelity is the degree to which the intervention was delivered as planned, rather than deviating from original design. Just as in other forms of intervention research, attention has to be paid to identifying the hypothesized effective ingredients of interventions and assessing the fidelity with which those intervention components are being delivered. For example, in a contact-based intervention the effective ingredients may be the scripted introduction, the description of the purpose, or the dialogue (Collins et al., 2012). The extent to which the quality of the interaction varies from the ideal model could pose one type of threat to internal validity and affect results (Shadish et al., 2002). Evans-Lacko and colleagues (2013b) reported on the active ingredients of a contact program delivered as part of the anti-stigma marketing campaign in England from 2009 to 2011. They found that personal contact predicted positive changes in knowledge and attitudes for the school students. Consumers' stories about their mental health problems and of their contact with a range of services had the greatest impact on the target audiences in terms of reducing mental illness stigma.

External Validity

Studies designed to understand social phenomena and to assess social interventions are often conducted with restricted populations (e.g., college students), which limits generalizability of the findings. Targeted and local stigma change has to be implemented and evaluated in real world settings to translate theory into practice and allow for more realistic tests of how, for example, employers in a large city or small town landlords respond to anti-stigma programs (Collins et al., 2012; Corrigan and Shapiro, 2010).

Cost-Benefit Analyses

Cost-benefit analyses are critically important in large national initiatives in which the return on investment is under scrutiny. As an example, data on the evaluation of the national Time to Change initiative in England (see Chapter 4) were combined with their social marketing campaign expenditure data to estimate the economic impact on employment for people with depression (Evans-Lacko et al., 2013a). Based on average national social marketing campaign costs, analysts found that the economic benefits outweighed costs and concluded that the campaign's anti-stigma social marketing component is a potentially cost-effective and low-cost intervention for reducing the impact of stigma on people with mental health problems. Canada is also incorporating economic analyses of workplace-based anti-stigma and mental illness awareness programs in their evaluations of the Opening Minds initiative (Pietrus, 2013). They are developing an economic model to estimate a breakeven point with the idea that stigma reduction may lead to reduction of a major source of disability costs (i.e., those from mental illness).

MONITORING NATIONAL TRENDS

In addition to evaluating the multiple interventions that constitute a national strategy for reducing stigma, resources also need to be invested in monitoring national trends in attitudes, beliefs, knowledge, and behaviors toward people with behavioral disorders. These trends need to be monitored to detect changes in structural, public, and self-stigma. Such trends would provide feedback loops on successful interventions or identify the possible need for course correction or new interventions. At present, for example, the United States lacks basic surveillance data and standards for reporting suicide and suicide attempts. This is one of the main challenges to the implementation of the National Strategy for Suicide Prevention (Caine, 2013). The rest of this section briefly suggests possible methods for monitoring changes in institutional structures (structural stigma), changes in social norms at the population level (public stigma), and changes in the lives of people who have been stigmatized including levels of self-stigma.

Monitoring Changes in Institutional Structures

Much research still needs to be carried out before measures of structural stigma can be operationalized and measured in order to monitor national trends. But there is promise in the methods being developed through studies conducted of:

- legislation and legal restrictions across many states, which document discrimination against people with mental illness (see, e.g., Burton, 1990; Corrigan et al., 2005b; Hemmens et al., 2002);
- discrimination suits filed under the Americans with Disabilities Act (ADA) for mental disorders (Colker, 2001; Scheid, 1999, 2005; Stuart, 2006);
- employment discrimination suits (Swanson et al., 2006); and
- disparity of funding for mental health services and research compared to general physical health (Kelly, 2006; Mark et al., 2014).

In addition, there are models from other countries. One example is how Canada is evaluating some of its initiatives to reduce sructural stigma by monitoring change in the media portrayals of peole with mental illness (the Media Monitoring Project) (Mental Health Commission of Canada, 2013).

Monitoring Changes in Social Norms at the Population Level

In earlier chapters, we presented findings from studies that examined social norms (public attitudes, beliefs, and behaviors) about people with mental and substance use disorders that prevail in the United States. Most survey items relating to stigma were added to surveys examining the prevalence of mental illness, substance use, or other conditions but were not necessarily carried out on a periodic basis. However, to monitor trends of a multipronged national initiative to reduce stigma, these types of items on population-based surveys would need to be re-administered on a periodic basis. Items would need to be reviewed and updated to capture the most recent research findings on indicators of stigma (e.g., attitudes, beliefs, behaviors, discrimination, access to care). The results would be important indicators of public health risk, in the same way as other contextual factors that are included on surveys (e.g., social support, housing, income, employment).

Several surveys could be considered as possible candidates if they could be administered on a regular periodic basis. For example, a mental health module of the General Social Survey (GSS) was administered in 1996 and repeated in 2006. As detailed in Chapter 2, substantial changes were seen over time in relation to respondents' understanding about mental illness and treatment (Pescosolido et al., 2010). Another example is the Behavioral Risk Factor Surveillance System (BRFSS) that incorporated a mental illness and stigma module in 2007 in which 35 states participated. Smaller numbers of states have participated in subsequent years because it is a voluntary add-on module to the BRFSS (Centers for Disease Control and Prevention et al., 2012). If these modules of the GSS or BRFSS were more broadly and continuously supported, they might be candidates for monitoring trends in public attitudes.

Another possible candidate is the National Survey of Drug Use and Health sponsored by the Substance Use and Mental Health Services Administration, which is administered annually and includes questions related to accessing services and unmet service needs. Respondents have a wide array of possible responses pertaining to reasons for not accessing services or treatments. Some of these reasons include stigma-related variables, such as concerns about confidentiality, potential negative opinions of neighbors and employers, and fear of being committed to a hospital. Differences from year to year in the numbers of people who access service, have unmet needs, and have reasons for not accessing services make this survey a candidate for monitoring trends in other attitudes, beliefs, and behaviors related to stigma.

Social media also have emerged as valuable resources for researchers collecting data on and monitoring trends in public attitudes and behaviors toward health. Twitter, in particular, has been used to track disease outbreaks, such as influenza, and also to successfully monitor suicide risk (Jashinsky et al., 2014). Due to the low cost and relative ease of use, researchers need to continue to explore social media platforms for monitoring behavioral health conditions, assessing public attitudes toward people with the conditions, and delivering anti-stigma messages (Jashinsky et al., 2014; Korda and Itani, 2013).

Monitoring Changes in the Lived Experience
of People Who Are Stigmatized

Monitoring changes in the lived experiences of people with mental and substance use disorders provides a ground-level view that would supplement results of monitoring changes in structural stigma and public stigma, as well as an evaluation of outcomes of anti-stigma campaigns or social inclusion interventions (Brohan et al., 2010).

Constructs of the lived experience of stigma include perceived public stigma, experienced and anticipated discrimination, self-devaluation, and stigma avoidance (Brohan et al., 2010; Luoma, et al., 2013), as well as more distal measures of the influence of stigma on treatment-seeking, relationships with family and friends, employment, and housing. As change in stigma would be measured over time, an ideal research design would be longitudinal. Repeated measure designs have been used to study stigma constructs, such as:

- the enduring effects of stigma on the well-being of men with dual diagnoses of mental disorder and substance abuse (Link et al., 1997);
- differences in the effects of court-ordered treatment versus no court order on stigmatization, symptoms, treatment engagement, self-esteem, quality of life, and functioning among people with serious mental illness (Link et al, 2008);
- whether psychological consequences of stigma associated with HIV are lasting or transitory (Kang et al., 2006);
- discrimination suits filed under ADA for mental disorders (Colker, 2001; Scheid, 1999, 2005; Stuart, 2006);
- employment discrimination suits (Swanson et al., 2006);
- the nature and variety of discrimination experiences in the community and their impact on self-stigma, psychosocial resources, and the course of illness (Wright et al., 2000); and
- disparity of funding between research for mental health services and research for general physical health (Kelly, 2006; Mark et al., 2014).

SUGGESTED AREAS FOR FUTURE RESEARCH

Although there is evidence in many areas of stigma research as summarized in earlier chapters of this report, critical gaps remain. For example, as described above, it should be a priority for the field to move beyond periodic surveys and develop a strategic plan for monitoring change on an ongoing basis in attitudes, beliefs, and behaviors at structural, public, and individual levels. Based on the information drawn from the public workshops, commissioned papers, and deliberations, the committee suggests areas for future stigma research in no order of priority, along with specific research questions related to these topical areas.

Stigma of Substance Use Disorders

Significantly more is known about the stigma of mental illness and related processes than about the stigma associated with substance use, abuse, and addiction. Surveys of public attitudes about multiple stigmatizing labels indicate that drug and alcohol misuse are viewed significantly more negatively than depression or schizophrenia (Schomerus et al., 2011). More research is needed on the nature, extent, and dynamics of stigma toward people with substance use disorders and the associated social- and psychological-related processes to better inform intervention and behavior change-related research. While some comparative stigma research suggests that there are common elements across stigmatized conditions (Fife and Wright, 2000; Pescosolido et al., 2010), more work is needed to identify the unique dimensions of stigma related to substance use disorders and what it has in common with mental illness and other stigmatizing conditions. Areas of future research might include

- What psychological, interpersonal, community, or social factors influence stigma toward people with substance use disorders are most amenable to change?
- Why is the public more stigmatizing of people with substance use disorders than people with mental illness?
- What is the role of cultural belief systems about health and illness related to stigma on substance disorders?
- Do people with co-occurring substance use and mental disorders experience stigma from multiple sources?
- Has criminalization of certain substance use worsened the impact of addiction on individuals and communities?
- Do 12-step programs diminish stigma? Do these programs promote shame, which worsens the impact of stigma?
- How do other public health approaches, such as harm reduction and "Housing First," interact with stigma prevention and reduction programs?
- What are the long-term outcomes of substance use disorder initiatives?

Reducing Structural Stigma

A large proportion of anti-stigma interventions have focused on public rather than structural stigma. Although there is also a dearth of research related to structural stigma, there is a relevant body of work examining the structural barriers that people with mental and substance use disorders face. Examples include discriminatory legislation that places restrictions on jury service, voting, holding political office, and parental custody rights; and health datasets that document negative outcomes of structural stigma on individuals, including treatment utilization, chronicity, or persistence of symptoms (e.g., Hatzenbuehler and Link, 2014; Hatzenbuehler et al., 2014). Studies are also needed to examine how structural, public, and self-stigma, interact with each other.

To fully address stigma at this level, research is needed to identify and target manifestations of structural stigma that are less easily recognized, such as the unintended consequences of anti-stigma efforts, and to understand how structural stigma persists in the presence of national legislative efforts to protect stigmatized groups such as parity laws (Corrigan et al. 2004b). Research is needed to clarify the impacts of new policies, along with their implementation and enforcement, on mental health and health-related disparities among people with behavioral health disorders.

The disproportionate representation of people with mental and substance use disorders in the criminal justice system is well established (e.g., Abramsky, 2015; Epperson and Pettus-Davis, 2015; Giliberti, 2015; Gingrich and Jones, 2015; Wisniewski, 2015). However, more research is needed to examine the relationships and pathways between criminality and the indicators of structural stigma and both criminal justice and health outcomes.

Additional Manifestations of Stigma

This section briefly identifies and defines manifestations of stigma that are not characterized as discrete in the same way that structural, public, and self-stigma are characterized in the research and intervention literature. These forms of stigma (label avoidance, double and intersecting stigmas, and courtesy or family stigma) require further study to understand their nature and role in the larger stigma complex, which have implications for new interventions.

Label Avoidance

The term "label avoidance" is related to both public and self-stigma. It occurs when people with behavioral disorders perceive stigma and opt to avoid the labeling it engenders by not seeking treatment or help that would identify them as a member of the stigmatized group (Abramsky, 2015; Corrigan et al., 2009a, 2014; Epperson and Pettus-Davis, 2015; Giliberti, 2015; Gingrich and Jones, 2015; Wisniewski, 2015). A systematic review by Clement and colleagues (2015) found that fear of the impact of disclosing one's mental or substance use disorder was the most commonly reported barrier to help-seeking. Label avoidance also undermines the outcomes of antidiscrimination legislation; for example, if an individual does not disclose to an employer, employment protections in the ADA, and its amendments, are not relevant (Cummings et al., 2013).

Results of a national survey examining the prevalence of mental disorders and treatment utilization found that approximately 10 percent of people who reported not seeking treatment avoided treatment for their disorders because they were afraid it would have negative impacts on neighbors and their jobs (Substance Abuse and Mental Health Services Administration [SAMHSA], 2013). Label avoidance and concerns about disclosure can also keep people from obtaining peer services and community support.

Double and Intersecting Stigmas

People with mental and substance use disorders such as HIV/AIDS may experience stigma related to other physical disorders, racial or ethnic heritage, sexual orientation, or gender identity. Gary (2005) used the term "double stigma" to describe the experience of mental illness across four ethnic minority groups in the United States. The author observed that the double stigma not only impeded treatment-seeking but may have contributed to the development of co-morbidities such as substance use disorders that might also go untreated.

In a qualitative study exploring the experiences of lesbian, gay, bisexual, and transgender (LGBT) individuals, Kidda and colleagues (2011) observed complex intersections of stigma experienced by the study participants in relation to mental illness and their LGBT identities. The resulting first-person narratives suggested that building supportive networks can smooth the path to resilience and recovery.

Courtesy or Family Stigma

Families and friends of individuals with mental and substance use disorders may experience a "courtesy" burden of stigma. Stigmatizing attitudes toward families of people with substance use disorders have been found to be greater than for other health conditions, and family members are more likely to be blamed for onsets and relapses of a relative's mental than physical disorder. These families were also more likely to say that they had been avoided socially by others (Corrigan et al., 2006a).

The experience of courtesy or family stigma can lead to self-stigma and self-blame, and it can undermine the support of friends and families for care-seeking (Corrigan et al., 2014). Public stigma also influences a family's previous experiences with treatment providers and with others in wider family and social circles. Hopeful beliefs about the possibility of recovery and positive attitudes toward people with mental illness and substance use disorders would encourage family members, neighbors, and friends to offer their support and encouragement.

Targeting and Evaluating Contact and Education Programs

There is robust evidence that contact is related to lower levels of stigma making contact-based interventions a prime strategy for implementing change. Optimal target groups for contact and education programs are those with influential roles in the lives of people with mental and substance use disorders (Corrigan, 2004, 2011). While targeted interventions have rightly addressed stigma in health care providers, law enforcement, journalists, and students, other important sources of stigma have seldom been sought out for research or interventions. These include landlords, religious leaders, policy makers, and human resources gatekeepers.

One potential, but largely untested, target group is government officials who often have influence over the funding of mental health and substance use treatment, the siting of treatment facilities, and the enactment and enforcement of laws and policies protecting (or harming) people with mental and substance use disorders.

Another target for research and intervention would be members of the criminal justice system in addition to law enforcement officers, including court officials and probation officers, all of whom have frequent contact with people with mental and substance use disorders, partly due to the criminalization of some substance use activity.

The media represent another potential target. Evaluations of interventions targeted at the media are sparse in the literature, and those that are published vary in quality (Borschmann et al., 2014; Clement et al., 2013; Corrigan, 2012). Social media, such as Facebook and Twitter, have been used in national efforts in Australia, New Zealand, Spain, and Sweden (Betton et al., 2015), but a comprehensive review was unable to identify interventions using multiple types of media or any that evaluated television, radio, cellphone, or movies (Clement et al., 2013).

Teachers and other lay advisors play important roles in promoting the mental health of children and adolescents and are another potential target for research and intervention. The public support for lay advisors such as teachers suggests that faith-based and community leaders are also potential audiences for contact-based intervention efforts, in particular, due to the supportive and affirmative role they have within their communities (Pescosolido et al., 2008a).

Emergency responders who are tasked with being the first on the scene in a wide range of crises could also be targets for anti-stigma interventions. Many people with substance use disorders receive their only treatment in the emergency room (Cohen et al., 2007; Pescosolido et al., 2008b).

Family and friends of people with mental and substance use disorders are among the most frequently cited perpetrators of discrimination in several national studies (Corker et al., 2013; Thornicroft et al., 2014), which suggests that research on and interventions tailored to these groups are essential elements of stigma change campaigns.

Children and adolescents are rarely targets of stigma change initiatives (Livingston, 2012). Peer-reviewed research on classroom anti-stigma programs for youth are particularly sparse in the literature (Mellor, 2014), although the Opening Minds initiative is currently evaluating several youth programs (Mental Health Commission of Canada, 2013). No media-based anti-stigma interventions for children have yet been fully evaluated (Clement et al., 2013).

In addition to research that identifies effective targets for interventions, more research is needed to understand the outcomes of contact and education programs, including internally valid hypothesis testing. Questions for future research might include

- How do outcomes of contact programs compare to education or combination (contact and education) programs?
- How do outcomes of contact and education programs compare to protest, advocacy, and legislative change strategies? Do they work in combination?
- Do early childhood, school-based stigma change initiatives influence the development of negative behavioral health social norms later in life?
- Given that many contact-based, anti-stigma initiatives come from within peer and activist communities, what are the factors that contribute to success of contact-based programs?

- What are the characteristics of peers who effectively deliver the desired message(s)?
- What are the most effective peer service training programs?

Measuring Behavior Change

Recent reviews of stigma change initiatives have found few studies that targeted and measured actual behavior toward people with mental illness (Dalky, 2012). As behavioral change is the ultimate goal of stigma reduction, more research efforts are required in this area. More and varied methods are needed for measuring behavior change in target populations because research suggests that greater awareness of mental illness or mental health literacy alone will not decrease stigma or discrimination against people with mental illness (Evans-Lacko et al., 2013b; Pescosolido, 2013; Schomerus et al., 2012).

In the broader prejudice and discrimination literature, the past 2 decades have seen a surge in the amount of work examining implicit measures of prejudice toward a wide range of social groups (Greenwald et al., 2009). People may hold automatic biases of which they are unaware that can in turn result in discriminatory behaviors that place people with substance use disorder at a disadvantage. Although these measures have received minimal attention in the stigma toward mental illness literature (O'Driscoll et al., 2012), they hold much promise to examine aspects of both self-stigma and public stigma, which are not necessarily accessible to one's conscious mental processes.

Finally, psychometric testing and validation of measures are needed within target populations and cannot be presumed to be generalizable based on strong reliability and validity in other populations (Brown, 2011).

The Stigma Complex

Much of what the literature suggests about influences on public stigma is theory based or speculative with little empirical backing. Even less is known about the development and predictors of self-stigma. This is due in part to the dearth of longitudinal research in this area (Kulesza et al., 2013). Robust longitudinal data would contribute to knowledge of stigma's antecedents and consequences, as well as the development of negative social norms over time in individuals and among the general public. Also important, longitudinal data would support efforts to monitor stigma change over time in the United States, including change across regions, and how change varies by demographic variables, such as sex, age, race, and ethnicity.

It would be important to follow the progress of successful anti-stigma initiatives in other countries, including the evolution of national norms and opinions over time, and specific knowledge gained about what changed public opinion, how long it took to effect change, and how the changes endure or continue to evolve in the desired direction(s).

Key issues to monitor in the United States include variability across states in implementation and enforcement of key legislation, including the ADA, Affordable Care Act, and Mental Health Parity Act and related outcomes for people with mental and substance use disorders.

Finally, research on stigma change efforts tend to focus on decreasing stigma and discrimination, but it is also important to monitor change in affirming attitudes and behaviors, for example, the belief that with proper support people with mental illnesses can perform and maintain jobs like people without mental illness (Corrigan and Shapiro, 2010).

Strategic Prioritization of Research

The topics above are not listed in order of priority since priorities change over time. SAMHSA will identify other research questions concerning its previous initiatives to improve behavioral health social norms.

SAMHSA has articulated its strategic *program* initiatives in areas of prevention of substance abuse and mental illness, health care and health systems integration, trauma and justice, recovery support, health information technology, and workforce development (Substance Abuse and Mental Health Services Administration, 2014). An important next step will be for SAMHSA to strategically prioritize *research* initiatives that will be informed by the science of changing behavioral health social norms.

A model for such prioritization of research was developed by the Transportation Research Board (2013). Although the methods were focused on transportation safety research, they can be applied across other fields. The overarching principles emphasize developing a data-driven approach of prioritization, encouraging collaboration and communication among stakeholders, encouraging bottom-up initiation of projects, joint funding to leverage resources for common purposes, focusing on "large, multi-modal research efforts of national importance" (Transportation Research Board, 2013, p. 8), and ensuring transparency of the prioritization process and results to all stakeholders.

The prioritization process includes several steps. Most important, the selection criteria need to be developed with a structure for weighting possible research projects. Considerations under this step include a project's contribution to the strategic vision; whether it has appropriate perspectives at the national, regional, or local level; how it fills a gap in the knowledge base; how it addresses an urgent or longer term needs; feasibility given existing resources, including the level of financial investment and risk; and potential value added in terms of economics, benefits to the end users, or support of other mission goals and objectives.

Subsequent steps involve publishing the selection criteria; developing a process for submitting proposals for future research projects; soliciting input from all stakeholders and all levels of organizations; developing a prioritized list of research projects that are based on the selection criteria and fit with mission, vision, and goals; and finally the identification of potential tradeoffs and alternate scenarios based on potential or varying levels of investments.

6

Conclusions and Recommendations

LESSONS LEARNED

Experiences of Other Countries

The experiences of Australia, Canada, and England (see Chapter 4) strongly indicate that changing negative social norms that stigmatize people with mental and substance use disorders will require a coordinated and sustained effort. Behavioral health-related norms and beliefs are created and reinforced at multiple levels, including day-to-day contact with people affected by mental and substance use disorders, organizational policies and practices, community norms and beliefs, the media, and governmental law and policy. Successful national-scale anti-stigma programs in other countries shared the following characteristics:

- They were supported by government at the national level.
- Support was committed on a long-term basis, often over decades.
- There was ongoing evaluation and monitoring from the planning phase forward.
- The initiative was multipronged to address the full range of relevant needs.
- Programs and services were coordinated across states (provinces) and across economic and social sectors to reduce fragmentation of efforts.

- Information was collected and disseminated about what worked, with whom, and under which conditions in order to inform the ongoing program development as well as future programs.

The Ryan White Act

In the United States, the Ryan White Care Act (RWCA) provides an example of a coordinated and sustained effort to meet the full spectrum of needs in people with HIV/AIDS. The act was initially passed by Congress in 1990 and has since been reauthorized four times in 1996, 2000, 2006, and 2009. The act supports programs and services at the community, municipal, and state level across the nation. Over the past 25 years, the Ryan White Program has become a critical component of the HIV/AIDS health care system in the United States, serving more than one-half million people (Crowley and Kates, 2013). The history, evolution, and outcomes of the program provide relevant information for future behavioral health anti-stigma initiatives.

The Ryan White Program has evolved to embrace a focus on treatment as prevention, which is consistent with the goals of the Affordable Care Act and the U.S. National HIV/AIDS Strategy. Ongoing evaluation and outcomes research provide future direction for the program, most recently in the areas of health workforce development, insurance coverage, and efforts to scale up programs to achieve population-level impacts (Crowley and Garner, 2015).

The Ryan White Program funds social support-related services in addition to traditional health care and prescription drug programs, including transportation and housing assistance, nutrition services, day care, and dental care (Taylor, 2010). Such "wrap-around" services are provided within the context of an integrated model of care to improve quality of life for people living with HIV/AIDS who face many of the stigma-related barriers as individuals with mental and substance use disorders (Garfield, 2011). Funding is awarded through statutorily established formula grants and through competitive mechanisms with the bulk of funds distributed noncompetitively in response to evolving needs.

One critique of RWCA is that the act did not establish minimum standards for care and services delivery across all states. For example, the act funded AIDS Drug Assistance Programs that were managed by individual states with the states deciding how to allocate funding and set eligibility for enrollment. At the program's peak height in September 2011, more than 9,000 people with HIV were on state medication waiting lists. Although state and local autonomy regarding implementation and delivery is essential, lessons learned from the AIDS Drug Assistance Programs underscore the need for unifying program standards and illustrate the important role of the federal government in a national strategy to reduce stigma related to mental and substance use disorders.

An Ecological Framework

Research on stigma toward mental and substance use disorders is challenging and complex in part because it necessarily involves a wide range of independent service systems, numerous sectors and professions, competing agendas, nuanced ethical and cultural issues, and multiple levels of outcome analysis ranging from the individual level to national statistics. Coordinating research across these many layers and systems will require a strategic and harmonious effort on the part of the federal government, private foundations, and academic and health care institutions, and other stakeholders. A coordinated research effort should be finely tuned to the societal and cultural contexts that intentionally or unintentionally endorse or facilitate stigma at various levels, especially the structural level. One assumption of an ecological perspective is that society's tolerance for or endorsement of a negative norm sets a precedent for stigma at the individual, family, and community levels (Institute of Medicine and National Research Council, 2014). This underscores the need to focus more attention on eliminating structural stigma (see Recommendation 2).

Understanding the processes by which factors at the individual, family, community, and social levels interact to produce and maintain stigma will require multidisciplinary, multimethod, and multisector approaches. Research will need to leverage and build on the existing knowledge base related to mental and substance use disorders, stigma change, and other relevant and related fields. Finally, effective research needs to consider the cultural processes, social stratification, ecological variations, and immigrant/acculturation status that are pertinent to understanding the causes and consequences mental and substance disorder stigma (Institute of Medicine and National Research Council, 2014. These sociocultural factors are critical elements to consider in developing and testing intervention strategies and in adapting evidence-based practices to unique populations and target audiences to ensure cultural relevance, reach, efficacy, and adoption (Barrera et al., 2013).

CONCLUSIONS AND RECOMMENDATIONS

A National-Level Approach

CONCLUSION: The experiences of the U.S. campaigns related to HIV/AIDS and of anti-stigma campaigns in Australia, Canada, and

England demonstrate the need for a coordinated and sustained effort over 2 or more decades to reduce the stigma associated with mental and substance use disorders.

Norms and beliefs related to behavioral health, such as the stigma associated with mental and substance use disorders, are created and reinforced at multiple levels, including day-to-day contact with affected individuals, organizational policies and practices, community norms and beliefs, the media, and governmental law and policy. A number of private and public organizations are already engaged in anti-stigma and mental health promotion efforts, but because these efforts are largely uncoordinated and poorly evaluated, they cannot provide an evidence base for future national efforts.

RECOMMENDATION 1: The U.S. Department of Health and Human Services should take the lead responsibility among federal partners and key stakeholders in the design, implementation, and evaluation of a multipronged, evidence-based national strategy to reduce stigma and to support people with mental and substance use disorders.

Relevant stakeholder groups would include the following:

- consumers in treatment for mental and substance use disorders and consumer organizations;
- families and others whose lives are touched by mental illness or substance use disorders, including suicide-attempt survivors and loss survivors;
- relevant private sector leadership, including major employers;
- relevant foundations and nongovernmental organizations;
- advocates and advocacy groups, including civil rights and disability law experts;
- insurance companies and pharmaceutical manufacturers;
- journalists and others in the news media, including public health media experts;
- health and behavioral health care providers, and administrators, including protective services and social services providers;
- health professional education institutions and professional associations;
- academic researchers, including suicide prevention experts and researchers;
- law enforcement officials and first responders; and
- representatives of federal, state, and local governments.

Early tasks would include the following:

- Identify a lead organization to serve as convener of stakeholders.
- Promote coordination and engagement across local, state, federal, and nongovernmental groups, including the U.S. Departments of Defense, Health and Human Services, Justice, and Labor, and relevant stakeholder groups to pool resources and promote evidence-based approaches.
- Evaluate current laws and regulations related to persons with mental and substance use disorders to identify opportunities to promote changes to support people on the path to recovery.
- Support the development of a strategic plan for research and dissemination of evidence about effective strategies to change social norms related to mental and substance use disorders (see Recommendation 3).
- With the federal agencies and other partners, develop a process of identifying and engaging grassroots efforts in each state to promote the implementation of evidence-based programs and fidelity monitoring of service delivery.
- With the federal agencies, establish a long-term, national monitoring system for stigma and stigma reduction.

Collaboration and Coordination

In 2013, eight federal agencies were identified as having programs to support individuals with mental and substance use disorders—the U.S. Departments of Defense, Education, Health and Human Services, Housing, Justice, Labor, Veterans Affairs, and the Social Security Administration—although their specific mission goals vary. To improve the effectiveness and extend the reach of the federal agencies' programs, there are some ongoing efforts to coordinate across the agencies and their programs (U.S. Government Accountability Office, 2014).

To maximize desired outcomes, collaborative efforts should eschew "ownership" of programs and include cobranding and resource sharing. The Substance Abuse and Mental Health Services Administration (SAMHSA's) ongoing engagement with stakeholders can support the search for common ground, mutually articulated goals, and shared agendas.

The committee has identified structural stigma and stereotypes of dangerousness and unpredictability as major sources of public and self-stigma. Given the importance of reducing stigma in these areas, early efforts could focus on development of a communications campaign that targeted policy and decision makers to challenge specific laws, policies and regulations that discriminate against people with mental and substance use disorders. Such a campaign could develop evidence-based public service announcements to hold in readiness for tragic events, such as mass violence, suicide by school and college students, and suicide clusters.

CONCLUSION: Changing stigma in a lasting way will require coordinated efforts, based on the best possible evidence, which are supported at the national level and planned and implemented by a representative coalition of stakeholders. Engaging a wide range of stakeholders would facilitate consensus building and provide the support needed to overcome major obstacles to the implementation of effective anti-stigma programs in the United States. Barriers and challenges include, but are not limited to, conflict among major stakeholder groups regarding best practices and priorities, resource constraints, and the need to target multiple audiences with variable perceptions and priorities, as well as shifting priorities at the national level.

RECOMMENDATION 2: The U.S. Department of Health and Human Services should evaluate its own service programs and collaborate with other stakeholders, particularly the criminal justice system and government and state agencies, for the purpose of identifying and eliminating policies, practices, and procedures that directly or indirectly discriminate against people with mental and substance use disorders.

Strategic Planning for Research

The committee defines strategic planning as the process undertaken by an agency or organization to define its future and formulate a detailed plan to guide its path from the current state to its vision for the future.

CONCLUSION: A planning process usually results in the development of a key document that includes a plan to ensure that communication is maintained across all stakeholders. This element is especially relevant for the Substance Abuse and Mental Health Services Administration given the agency's ongoing engagement with stakeholders and collaborators. A strategic plan can also serve as the basis of comparison for an ongoing plan for iterative effectiveness monitoring.

RECOMMENDATION 3: The Substance Abuse and Mental Health Services Administration should conduct formative and evaluative research as part of a strategically planned effort to reduce stigma.

SAMHSA's ongoing program of research on social norms and communications practices could coordinate with national efforts to achieve common goals and objectives. SAMHSA's Office of Communication's future activities could also be informed and supported by partners and participating stakeholders.

Because change occurs slowly, outcome evaluations need to be multifaceted and sustained to capture both direct and indirect effects, as well as intended and unintended consequences. An evaluation plan should include and support community-based participatory research that is based on the principle of partnership, in which community partners act as co-learners with academic partners rather than helpers and recipients. This approach involves community stakeholders in helping to define both the change targets and the intervention strategies, as well as in the conduct of the research itself. To inform a national campaign, more in-depth formative and evaluative research is critically needed in three areas: communication strategies, contact-based programs, and the role of peers.

Communication Strategies

Communication science provides a basis for understanding the effects of message features, contents, and platforms on four outcomes: cognitive (e.g., attention and memory), affective (e.g., liking, empathy, and fear), persuasive (e.g., attitude and behavior change), and behavioral (e.g., intents and actions). These effects are not discrete. They depend on characteristics of the target audience or audiences, the media platform, the message source, and the specific content and production features used in the message. For example, in a campaign to counter the stereotype of dangerousness in the wake of a tragic event, relevant audiences would include the media, school officials and teachers, young people, parents, and clergy. Messages would target specific smaller groups and would be designed and delivered with input and support of engaged stakeholders, for example, in donated airtime or volunteered time of high-profile supporters and speakers.

CONCLUSION: Best practices in choosing effective messages first require that a communications campaign develop well-defined goals for each specific group targeted. Effective messages can then be tailored to the specific target audience for the defined goals.

Because of the complexity of designing communication messages, efforts to implement the committee's recommendation on this topic should be informed by the results of formative and evaluative research. Research is necessary both before message concepts are generated and after message concepts are created for testing in the field. The perspectives of people with lived experience of mental and substance use disorders should inform anti-stigma campaigns at every stage, including design, delivery, and evaluation.

> **RECOMMENDATION 4: To design stigma-reduction messaging and communication programs, the Substance Abuse and Mental Health Services Administration should investigate and use evidence from formative and evaluative research on effective communication across multiple platforms.**

Several general features of effective communication programs have been identified by research and can inform the work in the committee's recommendations to SAMHSA:

- Identify specific target groups and specific goals appropriate to each group (e.g., legislators and policy makers, employers and landlords, educators, health care practitioners, and people with mental and substance use disorders).
- Make strong appeals that are relevant and personally consequential to particular audiences, for example, young people or veterans.
- Understand how a particular audience orients to a message and what kinds of cues and styles hold their attention so that the message is absorbed and remembered.
- Know what matters most to a specific target group.

Contact-Based Programs

Mixed-methods research has led to the identification of key elements of successful contact-based programs (Corrigan et al., 2013, 2014). Outcome research on contact demonstrates robust effects in pre-post studies (Corrigan et al., 2012; Griffiths et al., 2014) and at follow-up (Corrigan et al., 2015a). Although the efficacy of contact-based programs is greater than that of education programs alone in adults across a range of specific target audiences, such as health professionals, college students, and police, evidence shows that one-time contact is not as effective as repeated contact. Education programs are effective in changing stigmatizing attitudes among adolescents.

CONCLUSION: To expand the reach of contact-based programs, efforts will be needed to develop a nationally representative cohort of individuals who have disclosed information about their experiences of mental or substance use disorders. Involvement of those individuals needs to be preceded by the design of programs to aid personal consideration and action on disclosure decisions and of peer training programs to help people consider the risks and benefits of disclosure.

RECOMMENDATION 5: To decrease public and self-stigma and promote affirming and inclusive attitudes and behaviors targeted to specific groups, the Substance Abuse and Mental Health Services Administration should work with federal partners to design, evaluate, and disseminate effective, evidence-based, contact-based programming.

The Role of Peers

Peers play an essential role in combatting stigma, in part because they model personal recovery. Their role is critical in helping individuals to overcome the debilitating forces of self-stigma. Peer support programs and services include social and emotional support, as well as practical support related to quality-of-life decisions, delivered by people with mental and substance use disorders. Peer support has existed since the 1970s, but in 2001 several states began efforts to certify and train the peer specialist workforce. By 2012, 36 states had established such programs, although there is considerable variation in the certification programs across these states (Ostrow and Adams, 2012). State programs vary in terms of stage of development and certification requirements, including the content and process of training, examination criteria, and requirements for continuing education and recertification (Kaufman et al., 2012).

Most research on the outcomes of peer services has focused on quality-of-life measures. Few data are available about the costs and benefits of these programs, although the research suggests that people who use peer support services are more likely to use other behavioral health services of all kinds, including professional services and prescription drugs, which may lead to improved outcomes (Landers and Zhou, 2014). Although more peers are becoming certified, stakeholders disagree about the risks and benefits of professionalizing the role given grassroots origins of peer support in the consumer movement (Ostrow and Adams, 2012).

CONCLUSION: In the United States, there is no established and accepted set of national or state competencies or standards for peer

specialists, such as those that apply to other health professionals at state levels.

Although stakeholders do not agree on the risks and benefits of certification for peer support providers, it may contribute to the quality and outcomes of peer services and facilitate research on the effectiveness of these services across a range of outcomes. Programs need to be appropriately targeted to the audience or audiences and implemented at the relevant geographic level. Components of this effort would include standardization of preparation for peer service providers and development of practice guidelines for referral to and delivery of peer services across agencies and organizations engaged in this work. SAMHSA has taken steps in this direction with its 2009 *Consumer-Operated Service Evidence-Based Practices Toolkit* (Chapter 4) and continues to have an important role to play in the development and dissemination of these products and programs across the nation. The National Federation of Families for Children's Mental Health offers a national certification for parent support providers that could serve as a model for future efforts to expand the reach of high-quality peer support services.

> **RECOMMENDATION 6: The Substance Abuse and Mental Health Services Administration should work with partners to design, support, and assess the effectiveness of evidence-based peer programs to support people with mental and substance use disorders along the path to recovery and to encourage their participation in treatment.**

Development of a national strategy for eliminating the stigma of mental and substance use disorders is a challenging, long-term goal that will require collaboration across federal agencies, support from governments at all levels, and engagement of a broad range of stakeholders. No single agency can implement an effective national strategy, but SAMHSA brings specific and unique strengths including well-established stakeholder relations, commitment to the recovery model, and a history of promotion and implementation of prevention and early intervention strategies. Early objectives will include consensus building across a range of issues, design of cost-sharing arrangements, and development and implementation of a research strategy, including a system for monitoring change public attitudes, and mechanisms for disseminating information to inform future anti-stigma interventions.

References

Abramsky, S. (2015). One of the world's largest foundations is putting some real money into criminal justice reform. *The Nation*, April 28. Available: http://www.thenation.com/article/one-worlds-largest-foundations-putting-some-real-money-criminal-justice-reform/ [May 2016].

Abroms, L.C., and Maibach, E.W. (2008). The effectiveness of mass communication to change public behavior. *Annual Review of Public Health, 29,* 219-234.

Acosta, J., Martin, L.T., Fisher, M.P., Harris, R., and Weinick, R.M. (2012). *Assessment of the Content, Design, and Dissemination of the Real Warriors Campaign.* Santa Monica, CA: RAND.

Adam, D. (2013). Mental health: On the spectrum. *Nature, 496*(7446), 416-418.

Adlaf, E.M., Hamilton, H.A., Wu, F., and Noh, S. (2009). Adolescent stigma towards drug addiction: Effects of age and drug use behavior. *Addictive Behaviors, 34*(4), 360-364.

Ahmed, S.M., and Palermo, A.-G.S. (2010). Community engagement in research: Frameworks for education and peer review. *American Journal of Public Health, 100*(8), 1380.

Akabas, S.H., and Kurzman, P.A. (2005). *Work and the Workplace: A Resource for Innovative Policy and Practice.* New York: Columbia University Press.

Almond, D., Chay, K.Y., and Greenstone, M. (2006). *Civil Rights, the War on Poverty, and Black-White Convergence in Infant Mortality in the Rural South and Mississippi.* MIT Department of Economics Working Paper No. 07-04. Available: http://ssrn.com/abstract=961021 [March 2016].

American Foundation for Suicide Prevention. (2015*). Executive Summary: A Survey about Mental Health and Suicide in the United States.* Available: http://afsp.org/executive-summary-survey-mental-health-suicide-united-states/ [March 2016].

Andersen, R.M. (1995). Revisiting the behavioral model and access to medical care: Does it matter? *Journal of Health and Social Behavior, 36*(1), 1-10.

Anderson, L.M., Charles, J.S., Fullilove, M.T., Scrimshaw, S.C., Fielding, J.E., Normand, J., and Task Force on Community Prevention Services. (2003). Providing affordable family housing and reducing residential segregation by income: A systematic review. *American Journal of Preventative Medicine, 24*(3), 47-67.

Angermeyer, M.C., and Dietrich, S. (2006). Public beliefs about and attitudes toward people with mental illness: A review of population studies. *Acta Psychiatrica Scandinavica, 113*(3), 163-179.

Angermeyer, M.C., Schulze, B., and Dietrich, S. (2003). Courtesy stigma. *Social Psychiatry and Psychiatric Epidemiology, 38*(10), 593-602.

Angermeyer, M.C., Holzinger, A., Carta, M.G., and Schomerus, G. (2011). Biogenetic explanations and public acceptance of mental illness: Systematic review of population studies. *The British Journal of Psychiatry, 199*(5), 367-372.

Anthony, W.A. (2000). A recovery-oriented service system: Setting some system-level standards. *Psychiatric Rehabilitation Journal, 24*(2), 159-168.

Aoun, S., Pennebaker, D., and Pascal, R. (2004). To what extent is health and medical research funding associated with the burden of disease in Australia? *Australian and New Zealand Journal of Public Health, 28*(1), 80-86.

Arboleda-Flórez, J., and Stuart, H. (2012). From sin to science: Fighting the stigmatization of mental illnesses. *Canadian Journal of Psychiatry, 57*(8), 457-463.

Armstrong, M.L., Korba, A.M., and Emard, R. (1995). Of mutual benefit: The reciprocal relationship between consumer volunteers and the clients they serve. *Psychiatric Rehabilitation Journal, 19*(2), 45-49.

Atkin, C., and Freimuth, V. (1989). Guidelines for formative evaluation research in campaign design. In R.E. Rice and C. Atkin (Eds.), *Public Communication Campaigns* (pp. 53-69). Newbury Park, CA: Sage.

Barrera, M., Castro, F.G., Strycker, L.A., and Toobert, D.J. (2013). Cultural adaptations of behavioral health interventions: A progress report. *Journal of Consulting and Clinical Psychology, 81*(2), 196-205.

Barry, C.L., McGinty, E.E., Pescosolido, B.A., and Goldman, H.H. (2014). Stigma, discrimination, treatment effectiveness, and policy: Public views about drug addiction and mental illness. *Psychiatric Services, 65*(10), 1269-1272.

Bazelon Center for Mental Health Law. (2014). *When Opportunity Knocks . . . How the Affordable Care Act Can Help States Develop Supported Housing for People with Mental Illnesses.* Washington, DC: Author.

Betton, V., Borschmann, R., Docherty, M., Coleman, S., Brown, M., and Henderson, C. (2015). The role of social media in reducing stigma and discrimination. *The British Journal of Psychiatry, 206*(6), 443-444.

Bink, A.B. (2015). *Stigma and Discrimination in Behavioral and Physical Healthcare Settings.* Commissioned paper prepared for the Committee on the Science of Changing Behavioral Health Social Norms, August. Available: http://sites.nationalacademies.org/cs/groups/dbassesite/documents/webpage/dbasse_170041.pdf [May 2016].

Birnbaum, M.L., Candan, K., Libby, I., Pascucci, O., and Kane, J. (2014). Impact of online resources and social media on help-seeking behavior in youth with psychotic symptoms. *Early Intervention in Psychiatry.* doi: 10.1111/eip.12179.

Bischof, G., Rumpf, H.J., Meyer, C., Hapke, U., and John, U. (2005). Influence of psychiatric comorbidity in alcohol-dependent subjects in a representative population survey on treatment utilization and natural recovery. *Addiction, 100*(3), 405-413.

Bishop, T.F., Press, M.J., Keyhani, S., and Pincus, H.A. (2014). Acceptance of insurance by psychiatrists and the implications for access to mental health care. *Journal of the American Medical Association Psychiatry, 71*(2), 176-181.

Blair, J.P., and Schweit, K.W. (2013). *A Study of Active Shooter Incidents, 2000-2013.* Washington DC: Texas State University and Federal Bureau of Investigation, U.S. Department of Justice.

Bluthenthal, R.N., Kral, A.H., Gee, L., Erringer, E.A., and Edlin, B.R. (2000). The effect of syringe exchange use on high-risk injection drug users: A cohort study. *AIDS, 14*(5), 605-611.

Borinstein, A.B. (1992). Public attitudes toward persons with mental illness. *Health Affairs, 11*(3), 186-196.

Borschmann, R., Greenberg, N., Jones, N., and Henderson, R. (2014). Campaigns to reduce mental illness stigma in Europe: A scoping review. *Die Psychiatrie, 11*(1), 43-50.

Bos, A.E., Kanner, D., Muris, P., Janssen, B., and Mayer, B. (2009). Mental illness stigma and disclosure: Consequences of coming out of the closet. *Issues in Mental Health Nursing, 30*(8), 509-513.

Brohan, E., Slade, M., Clement, S., and Thornicroft, G. (2010). Experiences of mental illness stigma, prejudice and discrimination: A review of measures. *BMC Health Services Research, 10*(80), 1-11.

Brown, S.A. (2011). Standardized measures for substance use stigma. *Drug and Alcohol Dependence, 116*(1-3), 137-141.

Brown, S.A., Kramer, K., Lewno, B., Dumas, L., Sacchetti, G., and Powell, E. (2015). Correlates of self-stigma among individuals with substance use problems. *International Journal of Mental Health and Addiction, 13*(6), 687-698.

Burton, V.S. (1990). The consequences of official labels: A research note on rights lost by the mentally ill, mentally incompetent, and convicted felons. *Community Mental Health Journal, 26*(3), 267-276.

Busch, S.H., and Barry, C.L. (2008). New evidence on the effects of state mental health mandates. *Inquiry, 45*(3), 308-322.

Byrne, P. (2000). Stigma of mental illness and ways of diminishing it. *Advances in Psychiatric Treatment, 6*(1), 65-72.

Caine, E.D. (2013). Forging an agenda for suicide prevention in the United States. *American Journal of Public Health, 103*(5), 822-829.

Callard, F., Sartorius, N., Arboleda-Flórez, J., Bartlett, P., Helmchen, H., Stuart, H., Taborda, J., and Thornicroft, G. (2012). *Mental Illness, Discrimination and the Law: Fighting for Social Justice.* Hoboken, NJ: John Wiley & Sons.

Center for Behavioral Health Statistics and Quality. (2015). *Behavioral Health Trends in the United States: Results from the 2014 National Survey on Drug Use and Health.* HHS Publication No. SMA 15-4927, NSDUH Series H-50. Available: http://www.samhsa.gov/data/ [March 2016].

Centers for Disease Control and Prevention. (2015). *Injury Prevention and Control: Data and Statistics (WISQARS™).* Atlanta, GA: Author. Available: http://www.cdc.gov/injury/wisqars/ [March 2016].

Centers for Disease Control and Prevention, Substance Abuse and Mental Health Services Administration, National Association of County Behavioral Health and Developmental Disability Directors, National Institute of Mental Health, and the Carter Center Mental Health Program. (2012). *Attitudes Toward Mental Illness: Results from the Behavioral Risk Factor Surveillance System.* Atlanta, GA: Author.

Chandra, A., and Minkovitz, C.S. (2006). Stigma starts early: Gender differences in teen willingness to use mental health services. *Journal of Adolescent Health, 38*(6), 754.e1-754.e8.

Chinman, M., George, P., Dougherty, R.H., Daniels, A.S., Ghose, S.S., Swift, A., and Delphin-Rittmon, M.E. (2014). Peer support services for individuals with serious mental illnesses: Assessing the evidence. *Psychiatric Services, 65*(4), 429-441.

Chisolm, M.S., and Lyketsos, C.G. (2012). *Systematic Psychiatric Evaluation: A Step-By-Step Guide to Applying the Perspectives of Psychiatry.* Baltimore, MD: Johns Hopkins University Press.

Choe, J.Y., Teplin, L.A., and Abram, K.M. (2008). Perpetration of violence, violent victimization, and severe mental illness: Balancing public health concerns. *Psychiatric Services, 59*(2), 153-164.

Christison, G.W., and Haviland, M.G. (2003). Requiring a one-week addiction treatment experience in a six-week psychiatry clerkship: Effects on attitudes toward substance-abusing patients. *Teaching and Learning in Medicine, 15*(2), 93-97.

Clarke, D., Usick, R., Sanderson, A., Giles-Smith, L., and Baker, J. (2014). Emergency department staff attitudes towards mental health consumers: A literature review and thematic content analysis. *International Journal of Mental Health Nursing, 23*(3), 273-284.

Clay, R. (2013). Mental health first aid. *APA Monitor on Psychology, 44*(7), 32.

Clement, S., Lassman, F., Barley, E., Evans-Lacko, S., Williams, P., Yamaguchi, S., Slade, M., Rusch, N., and Thornicroft, G. (2013). Mass media interventions for reducing mental health-related stigma. *Cochrane Database of Systematic Reviews, 7,* Cd009453.

Clement, S., Schauman, O., Graham, T., Maggioni, F., Evans-Lacko, S., Bezborodovs, N., Morgan, C., Rüsch, N., Brown, J., and Thornicroft, G. (2015). What is the impact of mental health-related stigma on help-seeking? A systematic review of quantitative and qualitative studies. *Psychological Medicine, 45*(1), 11-27.

Cloud, D.H., Drucker, E., Browne, A., and Parsons, J. (2015). Public health and solitary confinement in the United States. *American Journal of Public Health, 105*(1), 18-26.

Cohen, E., Feinn, R., Arias, A., and Kranzler, H.R. (2007). Alcohol treatment utilization: Findings from the National Epidemiologic Survey on Alcohol and Related Conditions. *Drug and Alcohol Dependence, 86*(2), 214-221.

Colker, R. (2001). Winning and losing under the Americans with Disabilities Act. *Ohio State Law Journal, 62*. Available: http://ssrn.com/abstract=262832 [March 2016].

Collins, R.L., Wong, E.C., Cerully, J.L., Schultz, D., and Eberhart, N.K. (2012). *Interventions to Reduce Mental Health Stigma and Discrimination: A Literature Review to Guide Evaluation of California's Mental Health Prevention and Early Intervention Initiative.* Santa Monica, CA: RAND.

Collins, R.L., Wong, E.C., Roth, E., Cerully, J.L., and Marks, J. (2015). *Changes in Mental Illness Stigma in California during the Statewide Stigma and Discrimination Reduction Initiative.* Santa Monica, CA: RAND.

Colton, C.W., and Manderscheid, R.W. (2006). Congruencies in increased mortality rates, years of potential life lost, and causes of death among public mental health clients in eight states. *Preventing Chronic Disease, 3*(2), A42.

Cook, J.E., Purdie-Vaughns, V., Meyer, I.H., and Busch, J.T.A. (2014). Intervening within and across levels: A multilevel approach to stigma and public health. *Social Science and Medicine, 103,* 101-109.

Corbière, M., Zaniboni, S., Lecomte, T., Bond, G., Gilles, P.-Y., Lesage, A., and Goldner, E. (2011). Job acquisition for people with severe mental illness enrolled in supported employment programs: A theoretically grounded empirical study. *Journal of Occupational Rehabilitation, 21*(3), 342-354.

Corker, E., Hamilton, S., Henderson, C., Weeks, C., Pinfold, V., Rose, D., Williams, P., Flach, C., Gill, V., and Lewis-Holmes, E. (2013). Experiences of discrimination among people using mental health services in England 2008-2011. *The British Journal of Psychiatry, 202*(s55), s58-s63.

Corrigan, P.W. (2004). Target-specific stigma change: A strategy for impacting mental illness stigma. *Psychiatric Rehabilitation Journal, 28*(2), 113-121.

Corrigan, P.W. (2011). Best practices: Strategic stigma change (SSC): Five principles for social marketing campaigns to reduce stigma. *Psychiatric Services, 62*(8), 824-826.

Corrigan, P.W. (2012). Where is the evidence supporting public service announcements to eliminate mental illness stigma? *Psychiatric Services, 63*(1), 79-82.

Corrigan, P.W. (2014). Erasing stigma is much more than changing words. *Psychiatric Services*, 65(10), 1263-1264.

Corrigan, P.W. (2015). Challenging the stigma of mental illness: Different agendas, different goals. *Psychiatric Services*, 66(12), 1347-1349.

Corrigan, P.W., and Ben Zeev, D. (2012). Is stigma a stigmatizing word? A political question for science. *Stigma Research and Action*, 2(2), 62-66.

Corrigan, P.W., and Kleinlein, P. (2005). The impact of mental illness stigma. In P.W. Corrigan (Ed.), *On the Stigma of Mental Illness: Practical Strategies for Research and Social Change* (pp. 11-44). Washington, DC: American Psychological Association.

Corrigan, P.W., and Penn, D.L. (1999). Lessons from social psychology on discrediting psychiatric stigma. *American Psychologist*, 54(9), 765-776.

Corrigan, P.W., and Phelan, S.M. (2004). Social support and recovery in people with serious mental illnesses. *Community Mental Health Journal*, 40(6), 513-523.

Corrigan, P.W., and Rao, D. (2012). On the self-stigma of mental illness: Stages, disclosure, and strategies for change. *Canadian Journal of Psychiatry*, 57(8), 464.

Corrigan, P.W., and Shapiro, J.R. (2010). Measuring the impact of programs that challenge the public stigma of mental illness. *Clinical Psychology Review*, 30(8), 907-922.

Corrigan, P.W., River, L.P., Lundin, R.K., Penn, D.L., Uphoff-Wasowski, K., Campion, J., Mathisen, J., Gagnon, C., Bergman, M., Goldstein, H., and Kubiak, M.A. (2001). Three strategies for changing attributions about severe mental illness. *Schizophrenia Bulletin*, 27(2), 187-195.

Corrigan, P.W., Thompson, V., Lambert, D., Sangster, Y., Noel, J.G., and Campbell, J. (2003). Perceptions of discrimination among persons with serious mental illness. *Psychiatric Services*, 54(8), 1105-1110.

Corrigan, P.W., Watson, A.C., Warpinski, A.C., and Gracia, G. (2004a). Stigmatizing attitudes about mental illness and allocation of resources to mental health services. *Community Mental Health Journal*, 40(4), 297-307.

Corrigan, P.W., Markowitz, F.E., and Watson, A.C. (2004b). Structural levels of mental illness stigma and discrimination. *Schizophrenia Bulletin*, 30(3), 481-491.

Corrigan, P.W., Watson, A.C., Gracia, G., Slopen, N., Rasinski, K., and Hall, L.L. (2005a). Newspaper stories as measures of structural stigma. *Psychiatric Services*, 56(5), 551-556.

Corrigan, P.W., Watson, A.C., Heyrman, M.L., Warpinski, A., Gracia, G., Slopen, N., and Hall, L.L. (2005b). Structural stigma in state legislation. *Psychiatric Services*, 56(5), 557-563.

Corrigan, P.W., Watson, A.C., and Miller, F.E. (2006a). Blame, shame, and contamination: The impact of mental illness and drug dependence stigma on family members. *Journal of Family Psychology*, 20(2), 239-246.

Corrigan, P.W., Larson, J.E., Watson, A.C., Boyle, M., and Barr, L. (2006b). Solutions to discrimination in work and housing identified by people with mental illness. *Journal of Nervous and Mental Disease*, 194(9), 716-718.

Corrigan, P.W., Larson, J.E., and Ruesch, N. (2009a). Self-stigma and the "why try" effect: Impact on life goals and evidence-based practices. *World Psychiatry*, 8(2), 75-81.

Corrigan, P.W., Kuwabara, S.A., and O'Shaughnessy, J. (2009b). The public stigma of mental illness and drug addiction findings from a stratified random sample. *Journal of Social Work*, 9(2), 139-147.

Corrigan, P.W., Morris, S., Michaels, P.J., Rafacz, J.D., and Rüsch, N. (2012). Challenging the public stigma of mental illness: A meta-analysis of outcome studies. *Psychiatric Services*, 63(10), 963-973.

Corrigan, P.W., Kosyluk, K.A., and Rüsch, N. (2013). Reducing self-stigma by coming out proud. *American Journal of Public Health*, 103(5), 794-800.

Corrigan, P.W., Druss, B.G., and Perlick, D.A. (2014). The impact of mental illness stigma on seeking and participating in mental health care. *Psychological Science in the Public Interest, 15*(2), 37-70.

Corrigan, P.W., Michaels, P.J., and Morris, S. (2015a). Do the effects of antistigma programs persist over time? Findings from a meta-analysis. *Psychiatric Services, 66*(5), 543-546.

Corrigan, P.W., Bink, A.B., Fokuo, J.K., and Schmidt, A. (2015b). The public stigma of mental illness means a difference between you and me. *Psychiatry Research, 226*(1), 186-191.

Council of State Governments Justice Center. (2015). *Mentally Ill Offender Treatment and Crime Reduction Act Fact Sheet.* New York: Author. Available: https://csgjusticecenter.org/wp-content/uploads/2014/08/MIOTCRA_Fact_Sheet.pdf [March 2016].

Crisp, A.H., Gelder, M.G., Rix, S., Meltzer, H.I., and Rowlands, O.J. (2000). Stigmatization of people with mental illnesses. *The British Journal of Psychiatry, 177*(1), 4-7.

Crisp, A., Gelder, M., Goddard, E., and Meltzer, H. (2005). Stigmatization of people with mental illnesses: A follow-up study within the changing minds campaign of the royal college of psychiatrists. *World Psychiatry, 4*(2), 106.

Crowley, J.S., and Garner, C. (2015). *Aligning the Ryan White HIV/AIDS Program with Insurance Coverage.* Washington, DC: O'Neill Institute for National and Global Health Law-Georgetown Law.

Crowley, J.S., and Kates, J. (2013). *Updating the Ryan White HIV/AIDS Program for a New Era: Key Issues and Questions for the Future.* Washington, DC: Henry J. Kaiser Family Foundation.

Cummings, J.R., Lucas, S.M., and Druss, B.G. (2013). Addressing public stigma and disparities among persons with mental illness: The role of federal policy. *American Journal of Public Health, 103*(5), 781-785.

Cuthbert, B.N. (2014). The RDOC framework: Facilitating transition from ICD/DSM to dimensional approaches that integrate neuroscience and psychopathology. *World Psychiatry, 13*(1), 28-35.

Dalky, H.F. (2012). Mental illness stigma reduction interventions: Review of intervention trials. *Western Journal of Nursing Research, 34*(4), 520-547.

Davidson, L., Chinman, M., Kloos, B., Weingarten, R., Stayner, D., and Tebes, J.K. (1999). Peer support among individuals with severe mental illness: A review of the evidence. *Clinical Psychology: Science and Practice, 6*(2), 165-187.

Davis, J.K. (2010). Voting as empowerment practice. *American Journal of Psychiatric Rehabilitation, 13*(4), 243-257.

Deegan, P.E. (1992). The independent living movement and people with psychiatric disabilities: Taking back control over our own lives. *Psychosocial Rehabilitation Journal, 15*(3), 3-19.

DeParle, J. (1990). Rude, rash, effective, act-up shifts AIDS policy. *The New York Times.* January 3. Available: http://www.nytimes.com/1990/01/03/nyregion/rude-rash-effective-act-up-shifts-aids-policy.html?pagewanted=all [March 2016].

Desmarais, S.L., Van Dorn, R.A., Johnson, K.L., Grimm, K.J., Douglas, K.S., and Swartz, M.S. (2014). Community violence perpetration and victimization among adults with mental illnesses. *American Journal of Public Health, 104*(12), 2342-2349.

Diefenbach, D.L., and West, M.D. (2007). Television and attitudes toward mental health issues: Cultivation analysis and the third-person effect. *Journal of Community Psychology, 35*(2), 181-195.

Dolman, C., Jones, I., and Howard, L.M. (2013). Preconception to parenting: A systematic review and meta-synthesis of the qualitative literature on motherhood for women with severe mental illness. *Archives of Women's Mental Health, 16*(3), 173-196.

Downs, M.F., and Eisenberg, D. (2012). Help-seeking and treatment use among suicidal college students. *Journal of American College Health, 60*(2), 104-114.

Druss, B.G., Bradford, D.W., Rosenheck, R.A., Radford, M.J., and Krumholz, H.M. (2000). Mental disorders and use of cardiovascular procedures after myocardial infarction. *Journal of the American Medical Association, 283*(4), 506-511.

Dunion, L., and Gordon, L. (2005). Tackling the attitude problem. The achievements to date of Scotland's "See Me" anti-stigma campaign. *Mental Health Today,* 22-25.

Dunt, D., Robinson, J., Selvarajah, S., and Pirkis, J. (2010). *beyondblue: The National Depression Initiative 2005-2010 an Independent Evaluation Report.* Melbourne, AU: University of Melbourne.

Edney, D. (2004). *Mass Media and Mental Illness: A Literature Review.* Ontario: Canadian Mental Health Association.

Eiraldi, R.B., Mazzuca, L.B., Clarke, A.T., and Power, T.J. (2006). Service utilization among ethnic minority children with ADHD: A model of help-seeking behavior. *Administration and Policy in Mental Health and Mental Health Services Research, 33*(5), 607-622.

Eno Louden, J., and Skeem, J.L. (2013). How do probation officers assess and manage recidivism and violence risk for probationers with mental disorder? An experimental investigation. *Law and Human Behavior, 37*(1), 22-34.

Epperson, M., and Pettus-Davis, C. (2015). Reducing Illinois prison population is a marathon, not a sprint. *Chicago Sun Times.* April 10. Available: http://chicago.suntimes.com/news/7/71/514021/reducing-illinois-prison-population-marathon-sprint [March 2016].

Evans-Lacko, S., Brohan, E., Mojtabai, R., and Thornicroft, G. (2012a). Association between public views of mental illness and self-stigma among individuals with mental illness in 14 European countries. *Psychological Medicine, 42*(08), 1741-1752.

Evans-Lacko, S., London, J., Japhet, S., Rüsch, N., Flach, C., Corker, E., Henderson, C., and Thornicroft, G. (2012b). Mass social contact interventions and their effect on mental health related stigma and intended discrimination. *BMC Public Health, 12*(1), 489.

Evans-Lacko, S., Henderson, C., Thornicroft, G., and McCrone, P. (2013a). Economic evaluation of the anti-stigma social marketing campaign in England 2009-2011. *The British Journal of Psychiatry, 202*(s55), s95-s101.

Evans-Lacko, S., Malcolm, E., West, K., Rose, D., London, J., Rüsch, N., Little, K., Henderson, C., and Thornicroft, G. (2013b). Influence of time to change's social marketing interventions on stigma in England 2009-2011. *The British Journal of Psychiatry, 202*(s55), s77-s88.

Evans-Lacko, S., Corker, E., Williams, P., Henderson, C., and Thornicroft, G. (2014). Effect of the Time to Change anti-stigma campaign on trends in mental-illness-related public stigma among the English population in 2003-2013: An analysis of survey data. *The Lancet Psychiatry, 1*(2), 121-128.

Fazel, S., Gulati, G., Linsell, L., Geddes, J.R., and Grann, M. (2009). Schizophrenia and violence: Systematic review and meta-analysis. *PLoS Medicine, 6*(8), e1000120.

Ferguson, S.D. (1999). *Communication Planning: An Integrated Approach* (Vol. 1). Thousand Oaks, CA: Sage.

Fife, B.L., and Wright, E.R. (2000). The dimensionality of stigma: A comparison of its impact on the self of persons with HIV/AIDS and cancer. *Journal of Health and Social Behavior, 41*(1), 50-67.

Fineberg, N.A., Haddad, P.M., Carpenter, L., Gannon, B., Sharpe, R., Young, A.H., Joyce, E., Rowe, J., Wellsted, D., and Nutt, D. (2013). The size, burden, and cost of disorders of the brain in the UK. *Journal of Psychopharmacology, 27*(9), 761-770.

Foster, S.L., and Mash, E.J. (1999). Assessing social validity in clinical treatment research: Issues and procedures. *Journal of Consulting and Clinical Psychology, 67*(3), 308-319.

Frances, A.J., and Widiger, T. (2012). Psychiatric diagnosis: Lessons from the DSM-IV past and cautions for the DSM-5 future. *Annual Review of Clinical Psychology, 8,* 109-130.

Fu, K.-W., Cheng, Q., Wong, P.W., and Yip, P.S. (2015). Responses to a self-presented suicide attempt in social media. *Crisis, 34*(6), 406-412.

Fukkink, R. (2011). Peer counseling in an online chat service: A content analysis of social support. *Cyberpsychology, Behavior, and Social Networking, 14*(4), 247-251.

Gardner, E.M., McLees, M.P., Steiner, J.F., del Rio, C., and Burman, W.J. (2011). The spectrum of engagement in HIV care and its relevance to test-and-treat strategies for prevention of HIV infection. *Clinical Infectious Diseases, 52*(6), 793-800.

Garfield, R.L. (2011). *Mental Health Financing in the United States: A Primer.* Washington, DC: Henry J. Kaiser Family Foundation.

Gary, F.A. (2005). Stigma: Barrier to mental health care among ethnic minorities. *Issues in Mental Health Nursing, 26*(10), 979-999.

Gates, L.B., and Akabas, S.H. (2007). Developing strategies to integrate peer providers into the staff of mental health agencies. *Administration and Policy in Mental Health and Mental Health Services Research, 34*(3), 293-306.

Gates, L.B., Akabas, S.H., and Oran-Sabia, V. (1998). Relationship accommodations involving the work group: Improving work prognosis for persons with mental health conditions. *Psychiatric Rehabilitation Journal, 21*(3), 264-272.

Geller, G., Levine, D.M., Mamon, J.A., Moore, R.D., Bone, L.R., and Stokes, E.J. (1989). Knowledge, attitudes, and reported practices of medical students and house staff regarding the diagnosis and treatment of alcoholism. *Journal of the American Medical Association, 261*(21), 3115-3120.

Giacco, D., Matanov, A., and Priebe, S. (2014). Providing mental healthcare to immigrants: Current challenges and new strategies. *Current Opinion in Psychiatry, 27*(4), 282-288.

Giliberti, M. (2015). It's outrageous: Jails and prisons are no place to treat mental illness; just ask Paton Blough. *Huffpost Politics: The Blog.* May 21. Available: http://www. huffingtonpost.com/mary-giliberti/its-outrageous-jails-and-prisons-are-no-place-to-treat-mental-illness_b_7334026.html [March 2016].

Gingrich, N., and Jones, V. (2015). *Mental Illness Is No Crime.* Available: http://www.cnn. com/2015/05/27/opinions/gingrich-jones-mental-health/ [March 2016].

Gittelsohn, J., Steckler, A., Johnson, C.C., Pratt, C., Grieser, M., Pickrel, J., Stone, E.J., Conway, T., Coombs, D., and Staten, L.K. (2006). Formative research in school and community-based health programs and studies: "State of the art" and the TAAG approach. *Health Education & Behavior, 33*(1), 25-39.

Goffman, E. (1963). *Stigma: Notes on the Management of Spoiled Identity.* New York: Simon & Schuster.

Gould, M.S., Munfakh, J.L.H., Lubell, K., Kleinman, M., and Parker, S. (2002). Seeking help from the internet during adolescence. *Journal of the American Academy of Child & Adolescent Psychiatry, 41*(10), 1182-1189.

Grabe, M.E., Zhou, S., Lang, A., and Bolls, P.D. (2000). Packaging television news: The effects of tabloid on information processing and evaluative responses. *Journal of Broadcasting & Electronic Media, 44*(4), 581-598.

Graham, F.K. (1979). Distinguishing among orienting, defense, and startle reflexes. In H.D. Kimmel, E.H. Van Olst, and J.F. Orlebeke (Eds.), *The Orienting Reflex in Humans* (pp. 137–168). Hillsdale, NJ: Erlbaum.

Greenwald, A.G., Poehlman, T.A., Uhlmann, E.L., and Banaji, M.R. (2009). Understanding and using the implicit association test: III. Meta-analysis of predictive validity. *Journal of Personality and Social Psychology, 97*(1), 17-41.

Griffiths, K.M., Carron-Arthur, B., Parsons, A., and Reid, R. (2014). Effectiveness of programs for reducing the stigma associated with mental disorders. A meta-analysis of randomized, controlled trials. *World Psychiatry, 13*(2), 161-175.

Grob, G.N. (1991). *From Asylum to Community.* Princeton, NJ: Princeton University Press.

Grunig, J.E. (1989). Public audiences and market segments: Segmentation principles for campaigns. In C. Salmon (Ed.), *Information Campaigns: Balancing Social Values and Social Change* (pp. 199-228). Newbury Park, CA: Sage.

Harding, C., Brooks, G.W., Ashikaga, T., Strauss, J.S., and Breier, A. (1987a). The Vermont longitudinal study of persons with severe mental illness, I: Methodology, study sample, and overall status 32 years later. *American Journal of Psychiatry, 144*(6), 718-726.

Harding, C., Brooks, G.W., Ashikaga, T., Strauss, J.S., and Breier, A. (1987b). The Vermont longitudinal study of persons with severe mental illness, II: Long-term outcome of subjects who retrospectively met DSM-III criteria for schizophrenia. *American Journal of Psychiatry, 144*(6), 727-735.

Hart Research Associates. (2001). *The Face of Recovery.* Washington, DC: Author.

Hatzenbuehler, M.L., and Link, B.G. (2014). Introduction to the special issue on structural stigma and health. *Social Science & Medicine, 103*, 1-6.

Hatzenbuehler, M.L., O'Cleirigh, C., Grasso, C., Mayer, K., Safren, S., and Bradford, J. (2012). Effect of same-sex marriage laws on health care use and expenditures in sexual minority men: A quasi-natural experiment. *American Journal of Public Health, 102*(2), 285-291.

Hatzenbuehler, M.L., Bellatorre, A., Lee, Y., Finch, B.K., Muennig, P., and Fiscella, K. (2014). Structural stigma and all-cause mortality in sexual minority populations. *Social Science & Medicine, 103*, 33-41.

Hayes, S.C., Luoma, J.B., Bond, F.W., Masuda, A., and Lillis, J. (2006). Acceptance and commitment therapy: Model, processes, and outcomes. *Behavior Research and Therapy, 44*(1), 1-25.

Heflinger, C.A., and Hinshaw, S.P. (2010). Stigma in child and adolescent mental health services research: Understanding professional and institutional stigmatization of youth with mental health problems and their families. *Administration and Policy in Mental Health and Mental Health Services Research, 37*(1-2), 61-70.

Heijnders, M., and Van Der Meij, S. (2006). The fight against stigma: An overview of stigma-reduction strategies and interventions. *Psychology, Health & Medicine, 11*(3), 353-363.

Hemmens, C., Miller, M., Burton Jr, V.S., and Milner, S. (2002). The consequences of official labels: An examination of the rights lost by the mentally ill and mentally incompetent ten years later. *Community Mental Health Journal, 38*(2), 129-140.

Henderson, C., Noblett, J., Parke, H., Clement, S., Caffrey, A., Gale-Grant, O., Schulze, B., Druss, B., and Thornicroft, G. (2014). Mental health-related stigma in health care and mental health-care settings. *The Lancet Psychiatry, 1*(6), 467-482.

Hernandez, E.M., and Uggen, C. (2012). Institutions, politics, and mental health parity. *Society and Mental Health, 2*(3), 154-171.

Holman, L. (2011). Building bias: Media portrayal of postpartum disorders and mental illness stereotypes. *Media Report to Women, 39*(1), 12-19.

Hornik, R. (Ed.) (2002). *Public Health Communication: Evidence for Behavior Change.* London: Routledge.

Human Rights Watch. (2015). *Callous and Cruel: Use of Force Against Inmates with Mental Disabilities in U.S. Jails and Prisons.* Available: https://www.hrw.org/report/2015/05/12/callous-and-cruel/use-force-against-inmates-mental-disabilities-us-jails-and [March 2016].

Inciardi, J.A. (1986). *The War on Drugs: Heroin, Cocaine, Crime, and Public Policy* (Vol. 1). Palo Alto, CA: Mayfield.

Institute of Medicine. (2002). *Speaking of Health: Assessing Health Communication Strategies for Diverse Populations.* Committee on Communication for Behavior Change in the 21st Century: Improving the Health of Diverse Populations. Board on Neuroscience and Behavioral Health. Washington, DC: The National Academies Press.

Institute of Medicine. (2006). *Improving the Quality of Health Care for Mental and Substance-Use Conditions.* Committee on Crossing the Quality Chasm: Adaptation to Mental Health and Addictive Disorders. Washington DC: The National Academies Press.

Institute of Medicine and National Research Council. (2014). *New Directions in Child Abuse and Neglect Research.* Committee on Child Maltreatment Research, Policy, and Practice for the Next Decade: Phase II. A. Petersen, J. Joseph, and M. Feit (Eds.). Board on Children, Youth, and Families. Washington, DC: The National Academies Press.

James, D.J., and Glaze, L.E. (2006). *Mental Health Problems of Prison and Jail Inmates.* Washington, DC: U.S. Department of Justice, Office of Justice Programs, Bureau of Justice Statistics.

Jashinsky, J., Burton, S.H., Hanson, C.L., West, J., Giraud-Carrier, C., Barnes, M.D., and Argyle, T. (2014). Tracking suicide risk factors through twitter in the U.S. *Crisis, 35*(1), 51-59.

Jeffery, D., Clement, S., Corker, E., Howard, L.M., Murray, J., and Thornicroft, G. (2013). Discrimination in relation to parenthood reported by community psychiatric service users in the UK: A framework analysis. *BMC Psychiatry, 13*(1), 120.

Join Together. (2003). *Ending discrimination against people with alcohol and drug problems: Recommendations from a national policy panel.* Boston, MA: Join Together, Boston University School of Public Health.

Jorm, A.F. (2012). Mental health literacy: Empowering the community to take action for better mental health. *American Psychologist, 67*(3), 231-243.

Jorm, A.F., and Kitchener, B.A. (2011). Noting a landmark achievement: Mental health first aid training reaches 1% of Australian adults. *Australian and New Zealand Journal of Psychiatry, 45*(10), 808-813.

Jorm, A.F., and Reavley, N.J. (2014). Public belief that mentally ill people are violent: Is the USA exporting stigma to the rest of the world? *Australian and New Zealand Journal of Psychiatry, 48*(3), 213-215.

Jorm, A.F., Christensen, H., Griffiths, K.M., Jorm, A.F., Christensen, H., and Griffiths, K.M. (2005). The impact of beyondblue: The national depression initiative on the Australian public's recognition of depression and beliefs about treatments. *Australian and New Zealand Journal of Psychiatry, 39*(4), 248-254.

Jorm, A.F., Christensen, H., and Griffiths, K.M. (2006). Changes in depression awareness and attitudes in Australia: The impact of beyondblue: The national depression initiative. *Australian and New Zealand Journal of Psychiatry, 40*(1), 42-46.

Joseph, A.J., Tandon, N., Yang, L.H., Duckworth, K., Torous, J., Seidman, L.J., and Keshavan, M.S. (2015). #Schizophrenia: Use and misuse on Twitter. *Schizophrenia Research, 165*(2-3), 111-115.

Kang, E., Rapkin, B.D., and DeAlmeida, C. (2006). Are psychological consequences of stigma enduring or transitory? A longitudinal study of HIV stigma and distress among Asians and Pacific Islanders living with HIV illness. *AIDS Patient Care & STDs, 20*(10), 712-723.

Kaufman, L., Brooks, W., Steinley-Bumgarner, M., and Stevens-Manser, S. (2012). Peer specialist training and certification programs: A national overview. *University of Texas at Austin Center for Social Work Research, 10*, 07-011.

Keane, M. (1991). Acceptance vs. rejection: Nursing students' attitudes about mental illness. *Perspectives in Psychiatric Care, 27*(3), 13-18.

Keene, J.R. (2014). *Co-activation in the Motivational Systems and Motivational Inhibition: Processing and Emotional Judgments of Pictures and Framed Anti-Drug Messages.* Unpublished dissertation, Indiana University Bloomington.

Kelly, B.D. (2006). The power gap: Freedom, power and mental illness. *Social Science & Medicine, 63*(8), 2118-2128.

Khalifeh, H., Johnson, S., Howard, L., Borschmann, R., Osborn, D., Dean, K., Hart, C., Hogg, J., and Moran, P. (2015). Violent and non-violent crime against adults with severe mental illness. *The British Journal of Psychiatry, 206*(4), 275-282.

Kidd, S.A., Veltman, A., Gately, C., Chan, K.J., and Cohen, J.N. (2011). Lesbian, gay, and transgender persons with severe mental illness: Negotiating wellness in the context of multiple sources of stigma. *American Journal of Psychiatric Rehabilitation, 14*(1), 13-39.

Kilbourne, A.M., Keyser, D., and Pincus, H.A. (2010). Challenges and opportunities in measuring the quality of mental health care. *Canadian Journal of Psychiatry, 55*(9), 549-557.

Kim, H.S., Bigman, C.A., Leader, A.E., Lerman, C., and Cappella, J.N. (2012). Narrative health communication and behavior change: The influence of exemplars in the news on intention to quit smoking. *Journal of Communication, 62*(3), 473-492.

Kirby, S.D., Taylor, M.K., Freimuth, V.S., and Parvanta, C.F. (2001). Identity building and branding at CDC: A case study. *Social Marketing Quarterly, 7*(2), 16-35.

Klin, A., and Lemish, D. (2008). Mental disorders stigma in the media: Review of studies on production, content, and influences. *Journal of Health Communication, 13*(5), 434-449.

Knaak, S., Modgill, G., and Patten, S.B. (2014). Key ingredients of anti-stigma programs for health care providers: A data synthesis of evaluative studies. *Canadian Journal of Psychiatry, 59*(10 Suppl 1), S19-S26.

Koerting, J., Smith, E., Knowles, M., Latter, S., Elsey, H., McCann, D., Thompson, M., and Sonuga-Barke, E. (2013). Barriers to, and facilitators of, parenting programmes for childhood behaviour problems: A qualitative synthesis of studies of parents' and professionals' perceptions. *European Child & Adolescent Psychiatry, 22*(11), 653-670.

Korda, H., and Itani, Z. (2013). Harnessing social media for health promotion and behavior change. *Health Promotion Practice, 14*(1), 15-23.

Kranke, D., Floersch, J., Townsend, L., and Munson, M. (2010). Stigma experience among adolescents taking psychiatric medication. *Children and Youth Services Review, 32*(4), 496-505.

Kreuter, M.W., Green, M.C., Cappella, J.N., Slater, M.D., Wise, M.E., Storey, D., Clark, E.M., O'Keefe, D.J., Erwin, D.O., and Holmes, K. (2007). Narrative communication in cancer prevention and control: A framework to guide research and application. *Annals of Behavioral Medicine, 33*(3), 221-235.

Krieger, N., Rehkopf, D.H., Chen, J.T., Waterman, P.D., Marcelli, E., and Kennedy, M. (2008). The fall and rise of U.S. inequities in premature mortality: 1960-2002. *PLoS Medicine, 5*(2), e46.

Kulesza, M., Larimer, M.E., and Rao, D. (2013). Substance use related stigma: What we know and the way forward. *Journal of Addictive Behaviors, Therapy & Rehabilitation, 2*(2), 782.

Kummervold, P.E., Gammon, D., Bergvik, S., Johnsen, J.-A.K., Hasvold, T., and Rosenvinge, J.H. (2002). Social support in a wired world: Use of online mental health forums in Norway. *Nordic Journal of Psychiatry, 56*(1), 59-65.

Kvaale, E.P., Gottdiener, W.H., and Haslam, N. (2013a). Biogenetic explanations and stigma: A meta-analytic review of associations among laypeople. *Social Science & Medicine, 96,* 95-103.

Kvaale, E.P., Haslam, N., and Gottdiener, W.H. (2013b). The "side effects" of medicalization: A meta-analytic review of how biogenetic explanations affect stigma. *Clinical Psychology Review, 33*(6), 782-794.

Landers, G., and Zhou, M. (2014). The impact of Medicaid peer support utilization on cost. *Medicare & Medicaid Research Review, 4*(1), E1-E14.

Lang, A. (1989). Effects of chronological presentation of information on processing and memory for broadcast news. *Journal of Broadcasting & Electronic Media, 33*(4), 441-452.

Lang, A. (1990). Involuntary attention and physiological arousal evoked by structural features and emotional content in TV commercials. *Communication Research, 17*(3), 275-299.

Lang, A. (1995). Defining audio/video redundancy from a limited-capacity information processing perspective. *Communication Research, 22*(1), 86-115.

Lang, A. (2006). Using the limited capacity model of motivated mediated message processing to design effective cancer communication messages. *Journal of Communication, 56*(s1), S57-S80.

Lang, A., and Yegiyan, N.S. (2008). Understanding the interactive effects of emotional appeal and claim strength in health messages. *Journal of Broadcasting & Electronic Media, 52*(3), 432-447.

Lang, A., Geiger, S., Strickwerda, M., and Sumner, J. (1993). The effects of related and unrelated cuts on television viewers' attention, processing capacity, and memory. *Communication Research, 20*(1), 4-29.

Lang, A., Newhagen, J., and Reeves, B. (1996). Negative video as structure: Emotion, attention, capacity, and memory. *Journal of Broadcasting & Electronic Media, 40*(4), 460-477.

Lang, A., Zhou, S., Schwartz, N., Bolls, P.D., and Potter, R.F. (2000). The effects of edits on arousal, attention, and memory for television messages: When an edit is an edit can an edit be too much? *Journal of Broadcasting & Electronic Media, 44*(1), 94-109.

Lang, A., Borse, J., Wise, K., and David, P. (2002). Captured by the world wide web orienting to structural and content features of computer-presented information. *Communication Research, 29*(3), 215-245.

Lang, A., Park, B., Sanders-Jackson, A., and Wilson, B. (2007). Separating emotional and cognitive load: How valence, arousing content, structural complexity and information density affect the availability of cognitive resources. *Media Psychology, 10,* 317-338.

Lang, A., Kurita, S., Gao, Y., and Rubenking, B. (2013a). Measuring television message complexity as available processing resources: Dimensions of information and cognitive load. *Media Psychology, 16*(2), 129-153.

Lang, A., Sanders-Jackson, A., Wang, Z., and Rubenking, B. (2013b). Motivated message processing: How motivational activation influences resource allocation, encoding, and storage of TV messages. *Motivation and Emotion, 37*(3), 508-517.

Lang, A., Wu, Y., and Almond, A. (2014a). *Conceptualizing Combined Motivational Activation as the Mechanism Underlying Implicit Attitude Measurement.* Paper presented at the International Communication Association Communication Science Preconference. Seattle, Washington.

Lang, A., Schwartz, N., and Mayell, S. (2014b). Slow down you're moving too fast: Age, production pacing, arousing content, and memory for television messages. *Journal of Media Psychology: Theories, Methods, and Applications, 27*(2), 53-63.

Lang, A., Bailey, R.L., and Connolly, S.R. (2015). Encoding systems and evolved message processing: Pictures enable action, words enable thinking. *Media and Communication, 3*(1), 34-43.

Langford, L., Litts, D., and Pearson, J.L. (2013). Using science to improve communications about suicide among military and veteran populations: Looking for a few good messages. *American Journal of Public Health, 103*(1), 31-38.

Lawton, K.E., and Gerdes, A.C. (2014). Acculturation and Latino adolescent mental health: Integration of individual, environmental, and family influences. *Clinical Child and Family Psychology Review, 17*(4), 385-398.

Levey, S., and Howells, K. (1994). Accounting for the fear of schizophrenia. *Journal of Community & Applied Social Psychology, 4*(5), 313-328.

Lindberg, M., Vergara, C., Wild-Wesley, R., and Gruman, C. (2006). Physicians-in-training attitudes toward caring for and working with patients with alcohol and drug abuse diagnoses. *Southern Medical Journal, 99*(1), 28-35.

Link, B.G., and Phelan, J.C. (2001). Conceptualizing stigma. *Annual Review of Sociology, 27,* 363-385.

Link, B.G., Andrews, H., and Cullen, F.T. (1992). The violent and illegal behavior of mental patients reconsidered. *American Sociological Review, 57*(3), 275-292.

Link, B.G., Struening, E.L., Rahav, M., Phelan, J.C., and Nuttbrock, L. (1997). On stigma and its consequences: Evidence from a longitudinal study of men with dual diagnoses of mental illness and substance abuse. *Journal of Health and Social Behavior, 38*(2), 177-190.

Link, B.G., Phelan, J.C., Bresnahan, M., Stueve, A., and Pescosolido, B.A. (1999a). Public conceptions of mental illness: Labels, causes, dangerousness, and social distance. *American Journal of Public Health, 89*(9), 1328-1333.

Link, B.G., Monahan, J., Stueve, A., and Cullen, F.T. (1999b). Real in their consequences: A sociological approach to understanding the association between psychotic symptoms and violence. *American Sociological Review, 64*(2), 316-332.

Link, B.G., Yang, L.H., Phelan, J.C., and Collins, P.Y. (2004). Measuring mental illness stigma. *Schizophrenia Bulletin, 30*(3), 511-541.

Link, B.G., Castille, D.M., and Stuber, J. (2008). Stigma and coercion in the context of outpatient treatment for people with mental illnesses. *Social Science & Medicine, 67*(3), 409-419.

Livingston, J. (2012). Self-stigma and quality of life among people with mental illness who receive compulsory community treatment services. *Journal of Community Psychology, 40*(6), 699-714.

Livingston, J.D. (2013). *Mental Illness-Related Structural Stigma: The Downward Spiral of Systemic Exclusion.* Calgary, Alberta: Mental Health Commission of Canada. Available: http://www.mentalhealthcommission.ca [March 2016].

Livingston, J.D., Milne, T., Fang, M.L., and Amari, E. (2012). The effectiveness of interventions for reducing stigma related to substance use disorders: A systematic review. *Addiction, 107*(1), 39-50.

Livingston, J.D., Cianfrone, M., Korf-Uzan, K., and Coniglio, C. (2014). Another time point, a different story: One year effects of a social media intervention on the attitudes of young people toward mental health issues. *Social Psychiatry and Psychiatric Epidemiology, 49*(6), 985-990

Lloyd, C. (2013). The stigmatization of problem drug users: A narrative literature review. *Drugs: Education, Prevention, and Policy, 20*(2), 85-95.

Losen, D.J., and Welner, K.G. (2001). Disabling discrimination in our public schools: Comprehensive legal challenges to inappropriate and inadequate special education services for minority children. *Harvard Civil Rights-Civil Liberties Law Review, 36*(2), 407-460.

Luoma, J.B., O'Hair, A.K., Kohlenberg, B.S., Hayes, S.C., and Fletcher, L. (2010). The development and psychometric properties of a new measure of perceived stigma toward substance users. *Substance Use & Misuse, 45*(1-2), 47-57.

Luoma, J.B., Nobles, R.H., Drake, C.E., Hayes, S.C., O'Hair, A., Fletcher, L., and Kohlenberg, B.S. (2013). Self-stigma in substance abuse: Development of a new measure. *Journal of Psychopathology and Behavioral Assessment, 35*(2), 223-234.

Magliano, L., Fiorillo, A., De Rosa, C., Malangone, C., and Maj, M. (2004). Beliefs about schizophrenia in Italy: A comparative nationwide survey of the general public, mental health professionals, and patients' relatives. *Canadian Journal of Psychiatry, 49*(5), 322-330.

Maj, M. (2014). Keeping an open attitude towards the RDOC project. *World Psychiatry, 13*(1), 1-3.

Manago, B. (2015). *Understanding the Social Norms, Attitudes, Beliefs, and Behaviors Toward Mental Illness in the United States.* Commissioned paper prepared for the Committee on the Science of Changing Behavioral Health Social Norms. Available: http://sites. nationalacademies.org/cs/groups/dbassesite/documents/webpage/dbasse_170042. pdf [March 2016].

Mark, T.L., Levit, K.R., Yee, T., and Chow, C.M. (2014). Spending on mental and substance use disorders projected to grow more slowly than all health spending through 2020. *Health Affairs, 33*(8), 1407-1415.

Markowitz, F.E. (2001). Modeling processes in recovery from mental illness: Relationships between symptoms, life satisfaction, and self-concept. *Journal of Health and Social Behavior, 42*(1), 64-79.

Martin, J.K., Pescosolido, B.A., and Tuch, S.A. (2000). Of fear and loathing: The role of "disturbing behavior" labels and causal attributions in shaping public attitudes toward people with mental illness. *Journal of Health and Social Behavior, 41*(2), 208-223.

Martin, J.K., Pescosolido, B.A., Olafsdottir, S., and McLeod, J.D. (2007). The construction of fear: Americans' preferences for social distance from children and adolescents with mental health problems. *Journal of Health and Social Behavior, 48*(1), 50-67.

McGinty, E.E., Webster, D.W., and Barry, C.L. (2014). Effects of news media messages about mass shootings on attitudes toward persons with serious mental illness and public support for gun control policies. *American Journal of Psychiatry, 170*(5), 494-501.

McGinty, E.E., Goldman, H.H., Pescosolido, B., and Barry, C.L. (2015). Portraying mental illness and drug addiction as treatable health conditions: Effects of a randomized experiment on stigma and discrimination. *Social Science & Medicine, 126*, 73-85.

McLellan, A.T., Lewis, D.C., O'Brien, C.P., and Kleber, H.D. (2000). Drug dependence, a chronic medical illness: Implications for treatment, insurance, and outcomes evaluation. *Journal of the American Medical Association, 284*(13), 1689-1695.

McLeod, J.D., and Kaiser, K. (2004). Childhood emotional and behavioral problems and educational attainment. *American Sociological Review, 69*(5), 636-658.

Mechanic, D., McAlpine, D.D., and Rochefort, D.A. (2013). *Mental Health and Social Policy: Beyond Managed Care.* Upper Saddle River, NJ: Pearson Education.

Mellor, C. (2014). School-based interventions targeting stigma of mental illness: Systematic review. *The Psychiatric Bulletin, 38*(4), 164-171.

Melnychuk, R.M., Verdun-Jones, S.N., and Brink, J. (2009). Geographic risk management: A spatial study of mentally disordered offenders discharged from forensic psychiatric care. *International Journal of Forensic Mental Health, 8*(3), 148-168.

Mental Health Commission of Canada. (2013). *Opening Minds: Interim Report.* Calgary, Alberta: Mental Health Commission of Canada. Available: http://www.mentalhealthcommission.ca/English/system/files/private/document/opening_minds_interim_report. pdf [March 2016].

Meltzer, E.C., Suppes, A., Burns, S., Shuman, A., Orfanos, A., Sturiano, C.V., Charney, P., and Fins, J.J. (2013). Stigmatization of substance use disorders among internal medicine residents. *Substance Abuse, 34*(4), 356-362.

Metraux, S., Caplan, J.M., Klugman, D., and Hadley, T.R. (2007). Assessing residential segregation among Medicaid recipients with psychiatric disability in Philadelphia. *Journal of Community Psychology, 35*(2), 239-255.

Mojtabai, R. (2010). Mental illness stigma and willingness to seek mental health care in the European Union. *Social Psychiatry and Psychiatric Epidemiology, 45*(7), 705-712.

Moniz, M.H., Davis, M.M., and Chang, T. (2014). Attitudes about mandated coverage of birth control medication and other health benefits in a U.S. national sample. *Journal of the American Medical Association, 311*(24), 2539-2541.

Moorhead, S.A., Hazlett, D.E., Harrison, L., Carroll, J.K., Irwin, A., and Hoving, C. (2013). A new dimension of health care: Systematic review of the uses, benefits, and limitations of social media for health communication. *Journal of Medical Internet Research, 15*(4), e85.

Moses, T. (2010). Being treated differently: Stigma experiences with family, peers, and school staff among adolescents with mental health disorders. *Social Science & Medicine, 70*(7), 985-993.

Mowbray, C.T. (1997). *Consumers as Providers in Psychiatric Rehabilitation.* McLean, VA: International Association of Psychosocial Rehabilitation.

Muhlbauer, S. (2002). Experience of stigma by families with mentally ill members. *Journal of the American Psychiatric Nurses Association, 8*(3), 76-83.

Mukolo, A., Heflinger, C.A., and Wallston, K.A. (2010). The stigma of childhood mental disorders: A conceptual framework. *Journal of the American Academy of Child & Adolescent Psychiatry, 49*(2), 92-103.

Nairn, R., Coverdale, S., and Coverdale, J. (2011). A framework for understanding media depictions of mental illness. *Academic Psychiatry, 35*(3), 202-206.

National Alliance on Mental Illness. (2014). *State Mental Health Legislation 2014: Trends, Themes and Effective Practices.* Arlington, VA: Author

National Research Council. (2013). *Reforming Juvenile Justice: A Developmental Approach.* R.J. Bonnie, R.L. Johnson, B.M. Chemers, and J. Schuck, Editors. Committee on Assessing Juvenile Justice Reform. Committee on Law and Justice, Division of Behavioral and Social Sciences and Education. Washington, DC: The National Academies Press.

National Research Council. (2014a). *The Growth of Incarceration in the United States: Exploring Causes and Consequences.* Committee on Causes and Consequences of High Rates of Incarceration. J. Travis, B. Western, and S. Redburn (Eds.). Division of Behavioral and Social Sciences and Education. Washington, DC: The National Academies Press.

National Research Council. (2014b). *Implementing Juvenile Justice Reform: The Federal Role.* Committee on a Prioritized Plan to Implement a Developmental Approach in Juvenile Justice Reform. Committee on Law and Justice, Division of Behavioral and Social Sciences and Education. Washington, DC: The National Academies Press.

Nawková, L., Nawka, A., Adámková, T., Rukavina, T.V., Holcnerová, P., Kuzman, M.R., Jovanović, N., Brborović, O., Bednárová, B., Žuchová, S., Miovský, M., and Raboch, J. (2012). The picture of mental health/illness in the printed media in three central European countries. *Journal of Health Communication, 17*(1), 22-40.

Newhagen, J.E., and Reeves, B. (1992). The evening's bad news: Effects of compelling negative television news images on memory. *Journal of Communication, 42*(2), 25-41.

Niederkrotenthaler, T., Reidenberg, D.J., Till, B., and Gould, M.S. (2014). Increasing help-seeking and referrals for individuals at risk for suicide by decreasing stigma: The role of mass media. *American Journal of Preventative Medicine, 47*(3 Suppl 2), S235-243.

Noar, S.M. (2006). A 10-year retrospective of research in health mass media campaigns: Where do we go from here? *Journal of Health Communication, 11*(1), 21-42.

O'Driscoll, C., Heary, C., Hennessy, E., and McKeague, L. (2012). Explicit and implicit stigma towards peers with mental health problems in childhood and adolescence. *Journal of Child Psychology and Psychiatry, 53*(10), 1054-1062.

O'Keefe, D.J. (2013). The relative persuasiveness of different forms of arguments-from-consequences. In C.T. Salmon (Ed.), *Communication Yearbook* (vol. 36, pp. 109-135). New York: Routledge.

Olafsdottir, S., and Beckfield, J. (2011). Health and the social rights of citizenship: Integrating welfare state theory and medical sociology. In B. Pescosolido, J.K. Martin, J.D. McLeod and A. Rogers (Eds.), *Handbook of the Sociology of Health, Illness, and Healing: A Blueprint for the 21st Century* (pp. 101-115). New York: Springer.

Olsen, J.A., Richardson, J., Dolan, P., and Menzel, P. (2003). The moral relevance of personal characteristics in setting health care priorities. *Social Science & Medicine, 57*(7), 1163-1172.

Ostrow, L., and Adams, N. (2012). Recovery in the USA: From politics to peer support. *International Review of Psychiatry, 24*(1), 70-78.

Palamar, J.J., Kiang, M.V., and Halkitis, P.N. (2011). Development and psychometric evaluation of scales that assess stigma associated with illicit drug users. *Substance Use & Misuse, 46*(12), 1457-1467.

Papish, A., Kassam, A., Modgill, G., Vaz, G., Zanussi, L., and Patten, S. (2013). Reducing the stigma of mental illness in undergraduate medical education: A randomized, controlled trial. *BMC Medical Education, 13*(1), 141.

Parcesepe, A.M., and Cabassa, L.J. (2013). Public stigma of mental illness in the United States: A systematic literature review. *Administration and Policy in Mental Health and Mental Health Services Research, 40*(5), 384-399.

Parnas, J. (2014). The RDOC program: Psychiatry without psyche? *World Psychiatry, 13*(1), 46-47.

Pearson, M. (2015). *Stigma and Substance Use: A Methodological Review.* Commissioned paper prepared for the Committee on the Science of Changing Behavioral Health Social Norms. Available: http://sites.nationalacademies.org/cs/groups/dbassesite/documents/webpage/dbasse_170044.pdf [March 2016].

Peek, H.S., Richards, M., Muir, O., Chan, S.R., Caton, M., and MacMillan, C. (2015). Blogging and social media for mental health education and advocacy: A review for psychiatrists. *Current Psychiatry Reports, 17*(11), 88.

Perry, B.L. (2011). The labeling paradox stigma, the sick role, and social networks in mental illness. *Journal of Health and Social Behavior, 52*(4), 460-477.

Pescosolido, B.A. (2013). The public stigma of mental illness: What do we think; what do we know; what can we prove? *Journal of Health and Social Behavior, 54*(1), 1-21.

Pescosolido, B.A. (2015). The stigma complex. *Annual Review of Sociology, 41*, 87-116.

Pescosolido, B.A., Monahan, J., Link, B.G., Stueve, A., and Kikuzawa, S. (1999). The public's view of the competence, dangerousness, and need for legal coercion of persons with mental health problems. *American Journal of Public Health, 89*(9), 1339-1345.

Pescosolido, B.A., Martin, J.K., Link, B.G., Kikuzawa, S., Burgos, G., Swindle, R., and Phelan, J. (2000). *Americans' Views of Mental Illness and Health at Century's End: Continuity and Change.* Bloomington, IN: Consortium for Mental Health Services Research.

Pescosolido, B.A., Fettes, D.L., Martin, J.K., Monahan, J., and McLeod, J.D. (2007). Perceived dangerousness of children with mental health problems and support for coerced treatment. *Psychiatric Services, 58*(5), 619-625.

Pescosolido, B.A., Jensen, P.S., Martin, J.K., Perry, B.L., Olafsdottir, S., and Fettes, D. (2008a). Public knowledge and assessment of child mental health problems: Findings from the National Stigma Study-Children. *Journal of the American Academy of Child & Adolescent Psychiatry, 47*(3), 339-349.

Pescosolido, B.A., Martin, J.K., Lang, A., and Olafsdottir, S. (2008b). Rethinking theoretical approaches to stigma: A framework integrating normative influences on stigma (FINIS). *Social Science & Medicine, 67*(3), 431-440.

Pescosolido, B.A., Martin, J.K., Long, J.S., Medina, T.R., Phelan, J.C., and Link, B.G. (2010). "A disease like any other"? A decade of change in public reactions to schizophrenia, depression, and alcohol dependence. *American Journal of Psychiatry, 167*(11), 1321-1330.

Pescosolido, B.A., Medina, T.R., Martin, J.K., and Long, J.S. (2013). The "backbone" of stigma: Identifying the global core of public prejudice associated with mental illness. *American Journal of Public Health, 103*(5), 853-860.

Pettitt, B., Greenhead, S., Khalifeh, H., Drennan, V., Hart, T., Hogg, J., Borschmann, R., Mamo, E., and Moran, P. (2013). *At Risk, Yet Dismissed: The Criminal Victimisation of People with Mental Health Problems.* London: Victim Support, Mind.

Phelan, J.C. (2005). Geneticization of deviant behavior and consequences for stigma: The case of mental illness. *Journal of Health and Social Behavior, 46*(4), 307-322.

Phelan, J.C., Link, B.G., Stueve, A., and Pescosolido, B.A. (2000). Public conceptions of mental illness in 1950 and 1996: What is mental illness and is it to be feared? *Journal of Health and Social Behavior, 41*(2), 188-207.

Piat, M. (2000). The nimby phenomenon: Community residents' concerns about housing for deinstitutionalized people. *Health and Social Work, 25*(2), 127-138.

Pincus, H.A., and Fine, T. (1992). The "anatomy" of research funding for mental illness and addictive disorders. *Archives of General Psychiatry, 49*(7), 573-579.

Pugh, T., Hatzenbuehler, M.L., and Link, B. (2015). *Structural Stigma and Mental Illness.* Commissioned paper prepared for the Committee on the Science of Changing Behavioral Health Social Norms. Available: http://sites.nationalacademies.org/cs/groups/dbasse site/documents/webpage/dbasse_170045.pdf [March 2016].

Quinn, N., Knifton, L., Goldie, I., van Bortel, T., Dowds, J., Lasalvia, A., Scheerder, G., Boumans, J., Svab, V., Lanfredi, M., Wahlbeck, K., and Thornicroft, G. (2014). Nature and impact of European anti-stigma depression programmes. *Health Promotion International, 29*(3), 403-413.

Reavley, N.J., and Jorm, A.F. (2011). Stigmatizing attitudes towards people with mental disorders: Findings from an Australian national survey of mental health literacy and stigma. *Australian and New Zealand Journal of Psychiatry, 45*(12), 1086-1093.

Reeves, B., and Nass, C. (1996). *The Media Equation: How People Treat Computers, Television, and New Media Like Real People and Places.* Stanford, CA: CSLI.

Riley, G. (2011). Pursuit of integrated living: The fair housing act as a sword for mentally disabled adults residing in group homes. *Columbia Journal of Law and Social Problems, 45,* 177-224.

Rivera, A.V., DeCuir, J., Crawford, N.D., Amesty, S., and Lewis, C.F. (2014). Internalized stigma and sterile syringe use among people who inject drugs in New York City, 2010-2012. *Drug and Alcohol Dependence, 144,* 259-264.

Rogers, E.M., and Storey, J.D. (1987). Communication campaigns. In C. Berger and S. Chaffee (Eds.), *Handbook of Communication Science* (pp. 817-846). Newbury Park, CA: Sage.

Room, R. (2005). Stigma, social inequality, and alcohol and drug use. *Drug and Alcohol Review, 24*(2), 143-155.

Rosenfield, S. (1997). Labeling mental illness: The effects of received services and perceived stigma on life satisfaction. *American Sociological Review, 62*(4), 660-672.

Ross, C.A., and Goldner, E.M. (2009). Stigma, negative attitudes and discrimination towards mental illness within the nursing profession: A review of the literature. *Journal of Psychiatric and Mental Health Nursing, 16*(6), 558-567.

Salzer, M.S. (2012). A comparative study of campus experiences of college students with mental illnesses versus a general college sample. *Journal of American College Health, 60*(1), 1-7.

Sarteschi, C.M. (2013). Mentally ill offenders involved with the U.S. criminal justice system. *Sage Open, 3*(3). doi: 10.1177/2158244013497029.

Sartorius, N., Gaebel, W., Cleveland, H.R., Stuart, H., Akiyama, T., Arboleda-Flórez, J., Baumann, A.E., Gureje, O., Jorge, M.R., and Kastrup, M. (2010). WPA guidance on how to combat stigmatization of psychiatry and psychiatrists. *World Psychiatry, 9*(3), 131-144.

Scheid, T.L. (1999). Employment of individuals with mental disabilities: Business response to the ADA's challenge. *Behavioral Sciences & the Law, 17*(1), 73-91.

Scheid, T.L. (2005). Stigma as a barrier to employment: Mental disability and the Americans with Disabilities Act. *International Journal of Law and Psychiatry, 28*(6), 670-690.

Schiff, A.C. (2004). Recovery and mental illness: Analysis and personal reflections. *Psychiatric Rehabilitation Journal, 27*(3), 212-218.

Schneider, B. (2010). Housing people with mental illnesses: The discursive construction of worthiness. *Housing, Theory and Society, 27*(4), 296-312.

Schneider, E.F. (2004). Death with a story. *Human Communication Research, 30*(3), 361-375.

Schnittker, J. (2008). An uncertain revolution: Why the rise of a genetic model of mental illness has not increased tolerance. *Social Science & Medicine, 67*(9), 1370-1381.

Schomerus, G., and Angermeyer, M.C. (2008). Stigma and its impact on help-seeking for mental disorders: What do we know? *Epidemiologia e Psichiatria Sociale, 17*(01), 31-37.

Schomerus, G., Lucht, M., Holzinger, A., Matschinger, H., Carta, M.G., and Angermeyer, M.C. (2011). The stigma of alcohol dependence compared with other mental disorders: A review of population studies. *Alcohol and Alcoholism, 46*(2), 105-112.

Schomerus, G., Schwahn, C., Holzinger, A., Corrigan, P.W., Grabe, H.J., Carta, M.G., and Angermeyer, M.C. (2012). Evolution of public attitudes about mental illness: A systematic review and meta-analysis. *Acta Psychiatrica Scandinavica, 125*(6), 440-452.

Schraufnagel, T.J., Wagner, A.W., Miranda, J., and Roy-Byrne, P.P. (2006). Treating minority patients with depression and anxiety: What does the evidence tell us? *General Hospital Psychiatry, 28*(1), 27-36.

Schulze, B. (2007). Stigma and mental health professionals: A review of the evidence on an intricate relationship. *International Review of Psychiatry, 19*(2), 137-155.

Schulze, B., and Angermeyer, M.C. (2003). Subjective experiences of stigma. A focus group study of schizophrenic patients, their relatives, and mental health professionals. *Social Science & Medicine, 56*(2), 299-312.

The Sentencing Project. (2012). *Incarcerated Women.* Available: http://www.sentencing project.org/doc/publications/cc_Incarcerated_Women_Factsheet_Sep24sp.pdf [March 2016].

Shadish, W.R., Cook, T.D., and Campbell, D.T. (2002). *Experimental and Quasi-Experimental Designs for Generalized Causal Inference* (2nd Ed.). Independence, KY: Houghton Mifflin College Division.

Shera, W. (1996). Managed care and people with severe mental illness: Challenges and opportunities for social work. *Health & Social Work, 21*(3), 196-201.

Silins, E., Silins, E., Conigrave, K.M., Silins, E., Conigrave, K.M., Rakvin, C., Silins, E., Conigrave, K.M., Rakvin, C., and Dobbins, T. (2007). The influence of structured education and clinical experience on the attitudes of medical students towards substance misusers. *Drug and Alcohol Review, 26*(2), 191-200.

Sipe, T.A., Finnie, R.K., Knopf, J.A., Qu, S., Reynolds, J.A., Thota, A.B., Hahn, R.A., Goetzel, R.Z., Hennessy, K.D., and McKnight-Eily, L.R. (2015). Effects of mental health benefits legislation: A community guide systematic review. *American Journal of Preventative Medicine, 48*(6), 755-766.

Skiba, R.J., and Peterson, R.L. (2000). School discipline at a crossroads: From zero tolerance to early response. *Exceptional Children, 66*(3), 335-346.

Slater, M.D., Rouner, D., Domenech-Rodriguez, M., Beauvais, F., Murphy, K., and Van Leuven, J.K. (1997). Adolescent responses to TV beer ads and sports content/context: Gender and ethnic differences. *Journalism & Mass Communication Quarterly, 74*(1), 108-122.

Snyder, L.B., Hamilton, M.A., Mitchell, E.W., Kiwanuka-Tondo, J., Fleming-Milici, F., and Proctor, D. (2004). A meta-analysis of the effect of mediated health communication campaigns on behavior change in the United States. *Journal of Health Communication, 9*(sup1), 71-96.

Solomon, P. (2004). Peer support/peer provided services underlying processes, benefits, and critical ingredients. *Psychiatric Rehabilitation Journal, 27*(4), 392.

Sparks, J.V., and Lang, A. (2014). Mechanisms underlying the effects of sexy and humorous content in advertisements. *Communication Monographs, 82*(1), 134-162.

Stevelink, S.A.M., Wu, I.C., Voorend, C.G., and van Brakel, W.H. (2012). The psychometric assessment of internalized stigma instruments: A systematic review. *Stigma Research and Action, 2*(2).

Stuart, H. (2006). Mental illness and employment discrimination. *Current Opinion in Psychiatry, 19*(5), 522-526.

Stuart, H., and Sartorius, N. (2005). Fighting stigma and discrimination because of mental disorders. *Advances in Psychiatry, 2,* 79-86.

Stuart, H., Arboleda-Flórez, J., and Sartorius, N. (2012). *Paradigms Lost: Fighting Stigma and the Lessons Learned.* Oxford, UK: Oxford University Press.

Stuart, H., Chen, S.P., Christie, R., Dobson, K., Kirsh, B., Knaak, S., Koller, M., Krupa, T., Lauria-Horner, B., Luong, D., Modgill, G., Patten, S.B., Pietrus, M., Szeto, A., and Whitley, R. (2014a). Opening minds in Canada: Targeting change. *Canadian Journal of Psychiatry, 59*(10 Suppl 1), S13-S18.

Stuart, H., Chen, S.-P., Christie, R., Dobson, K., Kirsh, B., Knaak, S., Koller, M., Krupa, T., Lauria-Horner, B., and Luong, D. (2014b). Opening Minds: The Mental Health Commission of Canada's anti-stigma initiative. *Canadian Journal of Psychiatry, 59*(10 Suppl 1), S8.

Subramanian, R., Delaney, R.E., Roberts, S., Fishman, N., and McGarry, P. (2015). *Incarceration's Front Door: The Misuse of Jails in America.* New York: Vera Institute of Justice.

Substance Abuse and Mental Health Services Administration. (1999). *Mental Health: A Report of the Surgeon General.* Rockville, MD: Author.

Substance Abuse and Mental Health Services Administration. (2006). *National Consensus Statement on Mental Health Recovery.* Rockville, MD: Author.

Substance Abuse and Mental Health Services Administration. (2013). *Substance Abuse and Mental Health Services Administration, Results from the 2012 National Survey on Drug Use and Health: Summary of National Findings.* Rockville, MD: Author.

Substance Abuse and Mental Health Services Administration. (2014). *Leading Change 2.0: Advancing the Health of the Nation 2015-2018.* Rockville, MD: Author. Available: http://store.samhsa.gov/shin/content//PEP14-LEADCHANGE2/PEP14-LEADCHANGE2.pdf [March 2016].

Suzuki, L.K., and Calzo, J.P. (2004). The search for peer advice in cyberspace: An examination of online teen bulletin boards about health and sexuality. *Journal of Applied Developmental Psychology, 25*(6), 685-698.

Swanson, J.W., Burris, S., Moss, K., Ullman, M.D., and Ranney, L.M. (2006). Justice disparities: Does the ADA enforcement system treat people with psychiatric disabilities fairly? *Maryland Law Review, 66,* 94-139.

Swanson, J.W., McGinty, E.E., Fazel, S., and Mays, V.M. (2015). Mental illness and reduction of gun violence and suicide: Bringing epidemiologic research to policy. *Annals of Epidemiology, 25*(5), 366-376.

Taylor, J. (2010). *The Basics: The Ryan White Care Act.* Washington, DC: The National Health Policy Forum.

Teplin, L.A., McClelland, G.M., Abram, K.M., and Weiner, D.A. (2005). Crime victimization in adults with severe mental illness: Comparison with the national crime victimization survey. *Archives of General Psychiatry, 62*(8), 911-921.

Thornicroft, C., Wyllie, A., Thornicroft, G., and Mehta, N. (2014). Impact of the "Like Minds, Like Mine" anti-stigma and discrimination campaign in New Zealand on anticipated and experienced discrimination. *Australian and New Zealand Journal of Psychiatry, 48*(4), 360-370.

Thornicroft, G., Rose, D., and Kassam, A. (2007). Discrimination in health care against people with mental illness. *International Review of Psychiatry, 19*(2), 113-122.

Thorson, E., and Friestad, M. (1989). The effects of emotion on episodic memory for television commercials. In P. Cafferata and A.M. Tybout (Eds.), *Cognitive and Affective Responses to Advertising* (pp. 412-414). Lexington, MA: Lexington Books.

Torrey, E.F., Zdanowicz, M., Kennard, A., Lamb, H., Eslinger, D., Biasotti, M., and Fuller, D. (2014). *The Treatment of Persons with Mental Illness in Prisons and Jails: A State Survey.* Arlington, VA: Treatment Advocacy Center.

Tourangeau, R., and Yan, T. (2007). Sensitive questions in surveys. *Psychological Bulletin*, 133(5), 859.

Transportation Research Board. (2013). *National Cooperative Highway Research Program Report 756: Highway Safety Research Agenda: Infrastructure and Operations*. Washington, DC: Author.

Trujols, J. (2015). The brain disease model of addiction: Challenging or reinforcing stigma? *The Lancet Psychiatry*, 2(4), 292.

U.S. Government Accountability Office. (2014). *Mental Health: HHS Leadership Needed to Coordinate Federal Efforts Related to Serious Mental Illness*. GAO-15-113.Washington, DC: Author. Available: http://www.gao.gov/assets/670/667644.pdf [April 2016].

Van Boekel, L.C., Brouwers, E.P., Van Weeghel, J., and Garretsen, H.F. (2013). Stigma among health professionals toward patients with substance use disorders and its consequences for healthcare delivery: Systematic review. *Drug and Alcohol Dependence*, 131(1), 23-35.

Volkow, N.D., and Koob, G. (2015). Brain disease model of addiction: Why is it so controversial? *The Lancet Psychiatry*, 2(8), 677-679.

Wahl, O.F. (1999). Mental health consumers' experience of stigma. *Schizophrenia Bulletin*, 25(3), 467-478.

Wahl, O.F., Wood, A., and Richards, R. (2002). Newspaper coverage of mental illness: Is it changing? *Psychiatric Rehabilitation Skills*, 6(1), 9-31.

Wald, J., and Losen, D.J. (2003). Defining and redirecting a school-to-prison pipeline. *New Directions for Youth Development*, 2003(99), 9-15.

Wang, P.S., Demler, O., and Kessler, R.C. (2002). Adequacy of treatment for serious mental illness in the United States. *American Journal of Public Health*, 92(1), 92-98.

Webb, M., Burns, J., and Collin, P. (2008). Providing online support for young people with mental health difficulties: Challenges and opportunities explored. *Early Intervention in Psychiatry*, 2(2), 108-113.

Wei, Y., Hayden, J.A., Kutcher, S., Zygmunt, A., and McGrath, P. (2013). The effectiveness of school mental health literacy programs to address knowledge, attitudes and help-seeking among youth. *Early Intervention in Psychiatry*, 7(2), 109-121.

Weinreich, N. (1999). The "Don't Kid Yourself" Campaign Case Study. Excerpted from Weinreich, N. (1999) *Hands-on Social Marketing: A Step-by-Step Guide to Designing Change for Good*. Thousand Oaks, CA: Sage. Available: http://www.social-marketing.com/dky.html [May 2016].

Whiteford, H.A., Degenhardt, L., Rehm, J., Baxter, A.J., Ferrari, A.J., Erskine, H.E., Charlson, F.J., Norman, R.E., Flaxman, A.D., Johns, N., Burstein, R., Murray, C.J.L., and Vos, T. (2013). Global burden of disease attributable to mental and substance use disorders: Findings from the Global Burden of Disease Study, 2010. *The Lancet*, 382, 1575-1586.

Whitley, R., and Henwood, B.F. (2014). Life, liberty, and the pursuit of happiness: Reframing inequities experienced by people with severe mental illness. *Psychiatric Rehabilitation Journal*, 37(1), 68-70.

Wisniewski, M. (2015). Psychologist to head Chicago jail, nation's second largest. *Reuters*, May 29. Available: http://www.reuters.com/article/us-usa-chicago-prison-idUSKBN0O418T20150519 [March 2016].

Witte, K., and Allen, M. (2000). A meta-analysis of fear appeals: Implications for effective public health campaigns. *Health Education & Behavior*, 27(5), 591-615.

Wolff, N., Blitz, C.L., and Shi, J. (2007). Rates of sexual victimization in prison for inmates with and without mental disorders. *Psychiatric Services*, 58(8), 1087-1094.

Wright, A., Jorm, A.F., and Mackinnon, A.J. (2011). Labeling of mental disorders and stigma in young people. *Social Science & Medicine*, 73(4), 498-506.

Wright, E.R., Gronfein, W.P., and Owens, T.J. (2000). Deinstitutionalization, social rejection, and the self-esteem of former mental patients. *Journal of Health and Social Behavior, 41*(1), 68-90.

Xie, H. (2013). Strengths-based approach for mental health recovery. *Iranian Journal of Psychiatry and Behavioral Sciences, 7*(2), 5-10.

Yamaguchi, S., Wu, S.I., Biswas, M., Yate, M., Aoki, Y., Barley, E.A., and Thornicroft, G. (2013). Effects of short-term interventions to reduce mental health-related stigma in university or college students: A systematic review. *Journal of Nervous and Mental Disease, 201*(6), 490-503.

Yang, L.H., and Link, B. (2015). Measurement of attitudes, beliefs, and behaviors of mental health and mental illness. Commissioned paper prepared for the Committee on the Science of Changing Behavioral Health Social Norms. Available: http://sites.nationalacademies.org/cs/groups/dbassesite/documents/webpage/dbasse_170048.pdf [March 2016].

Yang, L.H., Purdie-Vaughns, V., Kotabe, H., Link, B.G., Saw, A., Wong, G., and Phelan, J.C. (2013). Culture, threat, and mental illness stigma: Identifying culture-specific threat among Chinese-American groups. *Social Science & Medicine, 88,* 56-67.

Yegiyan, N.S., and Yonelinas, A.P. (2011). Encoding details: Positive emotion leads to memory broadening. *Cognition & Emotion, 25*(7), 1255-1262.

Yeh, M., McCabe, K., Hough, R.L., Lau, A., Fakhry, F., and Garland, A. (2005). Why bother with beliefs? Examining relationships between race/ethnicity, parental beliefs about causes of child problems, and mental health service use. *Journal of Consulting and Clinical Psychology, 73*(5), 800.

Zillmann, D., and Brosius, H.-B. (2012). *Exemplification in Communication: The Influence of Case Reports on the Perception of Issues.* New York: Routledge.

Appendix A

Agendas: Public Workshops

Workshop #1
Lessons Learned from Diverse Efforts to Change Social Norms
March 18, 2015

This workshop is an activity of the Committee on the Science of Changing Behavioral Health Social Norms to assist the Substance Abuse and Mental Health Services Administration (SAMHSA) in its efforts to implement strategies that improve attitudes and beliefs about mental and substance use disorders. The workshop will explore lessons learned from previous media, communication, and other types of campaigns to change attitudes and behaviors in public health or other arenas. Workshop participants will explore design and outcomes of these campaigns including message development, platforms used for message delivery, targeted audiences, dose of the intervention (messaging), and related incentives. In discussions, we will examine the campaigns in terms of their attention to social determinants; degree of contact; and outcomes related to social inclusion, stakeholder engagement, and sustainability of change in social norms.

Wednesday, March 18

8:30   **WORKSHOP CHECK-IN**

9:00   **WELCOME FROM THE NATIONAL RESEARCH COUNCIL**
- Barbara Wanchisen, Director, Board on Behavioral, Cognitive, and Sensory Sciences

9:10   **WORKSHOP OVERVIEW AND GOALS**
- David Wegman, Committee Chair
- Lisa Vandemark, Study Director

9:30   **PANEL I ➜ Messaging**

Panel Synopsis: Lessons learned about messaging ("What you say") from previous efforts in relevant fields, about the importance of messaging in efforts to change social norms, including relevant elements of messaging, such as dimensionality, concept, definition, and structure

> **Moderator:** Joanne Silberner
> **Discussant:** Vicky Rideout, Committee Member
>
> **Panelists:**
> - *Key Principles in the Design of Effective Persuasive Messages: Engagement and Acceptance*—Joseph Cappella, Annenberg School for Communication
> - *Making the Most of Your Message: How Message Structure and Content Influence Attention, Cognition, Emotion, and Intentions*—Annie Lang, Indiana University
> - *Behavioral Economics and Social Marketing*—Tony Foleno, The Ad Council
> - *The Context and National Testing of PSAs: The "Schizo" Project*—Bernice Pescosolido, Indiana University

10:45   **BREAK**

11:00   *Remarks from SAMHSA*—Kana Enomoto, Deputy Administrator, SAMHSA

11:15   PANEL II → Methods

Panel Synopsis: This session will focus on exploring evidence-based platforms ("How you say it") that can be used for media/communications efforts, and the strengths and weaknesses of the various media types in the context of the social norms targeted for change.

> **Moderator:** Joanne Silberner
> **Discussant:** Bernice Pescosolido, Committee Member
>
> **Panelists:**
> * *Using Entertainment Media to Deliver Public Health Messages: A Case Study of Grey's Anatomy*—Vicky Rideout, VJR Consulting
> * *Reporting Mental Health Issues in a Rapidly Changing Media Landscape: Resources, New Developments, and Future Directions*—Rebecca Palpant Shimkets, The Carter Center
> * *National Advertising to Reduce Youth Tobacco Use: The Truth Campaign*—Donna Vallone, American Legacy Foundation

12:30   LUNCH

1:15   PANEL III → Big Picture Look at Social Change

Panel Synopsis: How did social norms on those issues change? What role did mass media campaigns play? What roles did other elements, such as public policy, regulatory changes, or grassroots campaigns play in influencing change in social norms?

> **Moderator:** Joanne Silberner
> **Discussant:** Rebecca Palpant-Shimkets, Committee Member
>
> **Panelists:**
> * *The Designated Driver Campaign*—Jay A. Winsten, Harvard University
> * *When You Know Better You Do Better*—Phill Wilson, Black AIDS Institute
> * *Legacy 2: Youth Smoking*—Robin Koval, American Legacy Foundation
> * *Gay & Lesbian Bullying Prevention*—Tony Foleno, The Ad Council

2:30   **PANEL IV → Case Studies in Changing Social Norms**

Panel Synopsis: Media and communications campaigns/strategies used to improve social norms, beliefs, and attitudes in health-related arenas in which negative social norms, chronicity, and behavior change are relevant (e.g., epilepsy, HIV/AIDS, cancer)

> **Moderator:** Joanne Silberner
> **Discussant:** William Holzemer, Committee Member

> **Panelists:**
> - *Epilepsy: Sources of Stigma and Campaign Efforts*: Joan Austin, Indiana University
> - *Reducing HIV-Related Stigma in Healthcare Settings: From Africa to Alabama*—Janet Turan, University of Alabama at Birmingham
> - *Deserve to Die: A Campaign That Uprooted Long-Held Beliefs*—Kay Cofrancesco, Lung Cancer Alliance

3:30   **BREAK**

3:45   **Reflections on Lessons Learned and Open Discussion**

Panel Synopsis: Discussants will reflect on panel presentations in the context of what we know about the effectiveness of different types of media and communications campaigns/strategies used to improve social norms, beliefs, and attitudes regarding mental and substance use disorder and access to treatment.

> **Moderator:** David Wegman

> **Panelists:**
> - Vicky Rideout, Committee Member
> - Bernice Pescosolido, Committee Member
> - Beth Angell, Committee Member
> - William Holzemer, Committee Member

4:30   **CONCLUDING COMMENTS**
- David Wegman, Committee Chair

4:45   **ADJOURN**

Workshop #2
Opportunities and Strategies to Promote
Behavior Change in Behavioral Health
April 15, 2015

Wednesday, April 15, 2015

8:00   **Workshop Check-in**

8:30   **Welcome from the National Research Council**
        Barbara Wanchisen, Director, Board on Behavioral, Cognitive,
        and Sensory Sciences

8:45   **Workshop Overview and Goals**
        Lisa Vandemark, Study Director
        David Wegman, Committee Chair

9:00   **Keynote Address**
        Alan I. Leshner
        CEO Emeritus, American Association for the Advancement of
        Science

9:30   **PANEL I → Domestic Perspectives**

Panel Synopsis: Panelists will present on successes and challenges
of U.S. national, state, and local campaign efforts aimed at changing
behavioral health social norms.

        Moderator: Judith Warner
        Discussant: Patrick Corrigan, Committee Member

        Panelists:
        • *Structural Stigma and the Health of Lesbian, Gay, and Bisexual
          Populations: Implications for Changing Social Norms*—Mark
          Hatzenbuehler, Columbia University.
        • *Peer Counselor: Wounded Healer Please Apply*—Peggy
          Swarbrick, Rutgers University
        • *Culture and How It Shapes and Protects Against Mental
          Illness Stigma: Empirical Illustrations from Chinese Groups*—
          Lawrence H. Yang, Columbia University
        • *The Role of Clinical Practitioners in Community and
          Institutional Promotion of Mental Health and Addiction
          Treatment: Toward Structural Competency*—Helena Hansen,
          New York University

10:45   BREAK

**11:00   PANEL II ➔ Implementing Change in the U.S. Context:
Critical Evaluations**

Panel Synopsis: How can SAMHSA implement change based on
evidence from previous campaigns?

> **Moderator:** Judith Warner
> **Discussant:** Beth Angell, Committee Member
>
> **Panelists:**
> * *CAMHSA*—Patrick Corrigan, Committee Member
> * *Results from a School-Based Intervention to Change Norms
>   About Mental Illnesses*—Bruce Link, Columbia University

12:00   LUNCH

**1:00   Presentation: A Cultural Cognitive Approach to
Communicating about Child Mental Health**

> **Presenter:** Nathaniel Kendall-Taylor, The Frameworks
> Institute
> **Moderator:** William Holzemer, Committee Member

**2:00   PANEL III ➔ Implementing Change in the U.S. Context:
Strategies for Reaching Audiences**

Panel Synopsis: Reflections on panel presentations in the context of
the lived experiences of consumers, advocates, family members, and
practitioners.

> **Moderator:** Rebecca Palpant Shimkets, Committee Member
>
> **Panelists:**
> * Clarence Jordan, Committee Member
> * Ruth Shim, Committee Member
> * Susan Rogers, National Mental Health Consumers' Self-
>   Help Clearinghouse
> * Joe Powell, Association of Persons Affected by Addiction

3:15   BREAK

3:30   **PANEL IV → Perspectives from Outside the United States**

Panel Synopsis: Panelists will present on successes and challenges of campaign efforts aimed at changing behavioral health social norms outside of the United States.

Moderator: Beth Angell, Committee Member
Discussant: Patrick Corrigan, Committee Member

Panelists:
- *Evaluation of England's National Time to Change Anti-stigma Campaign: Results from Phase One*—Sara Evans-Lacko, King's College, London
- *The Opening Minds Initiative of the Mental Health Commission of Canada*—Robert Edwards Whitley, McGill University
- *Changing Behavioral Health Social Norms: Interventions and Outcomes from Australia*—Anthony Jorm, University of Melbourne

4:45   **CONCLUDING COMMENTS**
- David Wegman, Committee Chair

5:00   **ADJOURN**

Appendix B

Biographical Sketches of Committee Members and Staff

David H. Wegman (*Chair*) is emeritus professor in the School of Health and Environment at the University of Massachusetts, Lowell, where he previously served as dean of the School of Health and Environment. He also serves as adjunct professor at the Harvard School of Public Health. His research focuses on epidemiologic studies across a range of health conditions, including respiratory disease, musculoskeletal disorders, and cancer. He has also written on public health and policy issues concerning hazard and health surveillance, methods of exposure assessment for epidemiologic studies, the development of alternatives to regulation, and the use of participatory methods to study occupational health risks. He is a national associate of the National Academies of Sciences, Engineering, and Medicine. He has a B.A. from Swarthmore College and an M.D. and an M.Sc. from Harvard University. He is board certified in preventive medicine (occupational medicine).

Beth Angell is associate professor in the School of Social Work at the Institute for Health, Health Care Policy, and Aging Research at Rutgers University. Her research focuses on serious mental illness, including predictors of treatment-seeking and treatment engagement and adherence; consumer-provider interactions and relationships; and mandated treatment. Her current projects focus on vulnerable populations, including incarcerated persons and those with serious and persistent mental illness. She has an M.S.S.W. and a Ph.D. in social welfare from the University of Wisconsin–Madison.

Joseph N. Cappella is the Gerald R. Miller professor of communication at the Annenberg School for Communication at the University of Pennsylvania. His research areas include social cognition, communication theory, health communication, persuasion and politics, nonverbal behavior, and statistical and mathematical methods. He also conducts studies on cognitive processing of verbal and visual materials, organization of social interaction, and message effects. His book with Kathleen Hall Jamieson on the spiral of cynicism has won prizes from the American Political Science Association and the International Communications Association. He is a fellow of the International Communication Association, a past president, and a recipient of its B. Aubrey Fisher Mentorship Award. He is also a distinguished scholar of the National Communication Association. He has a Ph.D. in communication from Michigan State University.

Patrick Corrigan is distinguished professor of psychology at the Illinois Institute of Technology. Previously, he was associate dean for research in the Institute of Psychology at Illinois Institute of Technology and professor of psychiatry at the Northwestern University Feinberg School of Medicine and at the Pritzker School of Medicine at the University of Chicago. His research examines psychiatric disability and the impact of stigma on recovery and rehabilitation. Currently, he is principal investigator of the National Consortium for Stigma and Empowerment, a collaboration of investigators from more than a dozen research institutions. He has a Psy.D. in clinical psychology from the Illinois School of Professional Psychology.

William L. Holzemer is dean and distinguished professor of nursing at Rutgers University. Previously, he was associate dean for research and chair of the Department of Community Health Systems at the School of Nursing at the University of California, San Francisco. His research has focused on living well with HIV/AIDS, including the aspects of adherence, stigma, symptoms, and quality of life. He recently completed studies exploring the impact of HIV stigma on quality of care for people living with HIV infection in five African nations. He is a member of the National Academy of Medicine (formerly the Institute of Medicine). He has a B.S. in nursing from San Francisco State University and a Ph.D. in education from Syracuse University.

Clarence Jordan is vice president of wellness and recovery at Value Options, Inc., where he leads a multidisciplinary team devoted to providing recovery-based services, including a network of peers who work directly with adults and families. Previously, he was manager of the consumer recovery services for Magellan Health Services, Inc. He has held various positions with the National Alliance on Mental Illness at both the state and national levels, including serving as vice chair of its Veterans Committee and a member of its National African American Leaders Group and Multicultural Action Committee, working to improve outreach initiatives to the African American community. His work focuses on peer specialist services, wellness and recovery, and the stigma of mental illness and substance abuse. He is a recipient of the Consumer Leadership Award of the Substance Abuse and Mental Health Services Administration. He has an M.B.A. from the Naval Postgraduate School and an M.S. from the University of Arkansas, Fayetteville.

Annie Lang is distinguished professor of telecommunications and cognitive science at Indiana University. Her research seeks to explain how people process mediated messages, and she has developed a general data-driven model of mediated message processing. She is a fellow of the International Communication Association and a recipient of its Steven H. Chaffee Career Productivity Award. She has a Ph.D. in mass communication from the University of Wisconsin–Madison.

Vanessa Lazar (*Research Associate*) is on the staff of the National Academies of Sciences, Engineering, and Medicine. Her other recent work has included a study assessing intrapersonal and interpersonal competencies and on the Academies Gulf Research Program. Previously, she was a science assistant at the National Science Foundation in the Division of Behavioral and Cognitive Sciences and a research assistant at Brown University. She has a B.A. in psychology and an M.A. in marine affairs from the University of Rhode Island.

Bernice A. Pescosolido is distinguished professor of sociology at Indiana University and director of the Indiana Consortium for Mental Health Services Research. Her research addresses how social networks connect individuals to their communities and to institutional structures, providing the "wires" through which people's attitudes and actions are influenced. She has led teams of researchers on a series of national and international stigma studies, including the first U.S. national study in 40 years, the first national study of children's mental health, and the first global study of 16 countries representing all six inhabited continents. She is the recipient of numerous career, scientific, and community awards, including the Wilbur Lucius Cross Medal from Yale University, the Carl A. Taube Award for Distinguished Contributions to the Field of Mental Health Services Research from the Mental Health Section of the American Public Health Association, and the Leonard I. Pearlin Award for Distinguished Contributions to the Sociological Study of Mental Health from the American

Sociological Association. She has an M.A., an M.Phil., and a Ph.D. in sociology from Yale University.

Jeanne C. Rivard (*Senior Program Officer*) is on the staff of the National Academies of Sciences, Engineering, and Medicine. Most recently, she served as the study director of a major project on proposed changes to federal regulations for protecting human participants in research and the costudy director of an evaluation of the National Institute on Disability and Rehabilitation Research and its grantees. Previously, she was with the National Association of State Mental Health Program Directors Research Institute and on the faculty of the Columbia University School of Social Work. Her work has focused on interagency collaboration and evaluation of mental health services and trauma interventions. She has an M.S.W. from the University of South Carolina and a Ph.D. in social work from the University of North Carolina at Chapel Hill.

Ruth Shim is vice chair of education and faculty development in the Department of Psychiatry at Lenox Hill Hospital in New York City. Formerly, she was an associate professor in the Department of Psychiatry and Behavioral Sciences at Morehouse School of Medicine and the associate director of behavioral health at the National Center for Primary Care. Her research interests include mental health stigma, integration of primary care and behavioral health care, and mental health disparities. She has ongoing collaborative relationships with the Carter Center Mental Health Program, the Satcher Health Leadership Institute at Morehouse School of Medicine, and the Center for Behavioral Health Policy Studies at the Rollins School of Public Health at Emory University. She is a fellow of the American Psychiatric Association and is a member of the Preventive Psychiatry Committee and the Fellowship Committee of the Group for the Advancement of Psychiatry. She has an M.P.H. in health policy and an M.D. from Emory University.

Rebecca Palpant Shimkets is assistant director for the Rosalynn Carter Fellowships for Mental Health Journalism of the Carter Center Mental Health Program at Emory University. In that position, she developed and oversees a journalism fellowship program that each year awards stipends to 10 professional journalists in the United States, Romania, and Colombia to produce a significant work on mental health or mental illnesses. She is also responsible for designing new initiatives related to stigma reduction and measurement and advising on programming, including the annual national symposium and a program for new initiative development at the center. She is an active participant on advisory boards and in national work groups related to stigma and accurate portrayals of mental illnesses in the media. She has an M.S. in community counseling from Georgia State University.

Lisa M. Vandemark (*Study Director*) is a senior program officer at the National Academies of Sciences, Engineering, and Medicine. She is also a psychiatric nurse practitioner in the District of Columbia, working with children and families and adjunct faculty in the Department of Acute and Chronic Care at Johns Hopkins University School of Nursing. Her previous studies focused primarily on social and environment influences on health and health outcomes in the United States and in developing countries. Previously, she was on the faculty at the Medical University of South Carolina, where she taught in the psychiatric nurse practitioner and global health programs. She has a master's degree in psychiatric nursing from Rush University and a Ph.D. in geography from Rutgers University.

Eric R. Wright is professor of sociology and public health at Georgia State University and a Second Century Initiative faculty in the university's Atlanta Census Research Data-Health Policy and Risky Behaviors Cluster. Previously, he was a professor and chair of the Department of Health Policy and Management and director of the Center for Health Policy at the Richard M. Fairbanks School of Public Health at Indiana University-Purdue University Indianapolis. As a medical sociologist, his research interests center on social and public policy responses to mental health and illness, substance use and addictions, sexual health, and HIV/STI prevention. His research focuses on understanding and ameliorating health problems and disparities in minority and other vulnerable communities, including lesbian, gay, bisexual, and transgender people. He also works with community organizations and local and state governments to better understand community health needs and improve the effectiveness of health- and health care-related programs and policies. He has an M.A. and a Ph.D. in sociology from Indiana University, Bloomington.